CONTENTS

GOOD SEX

Jim Hancock and Kara Eckmann Powell

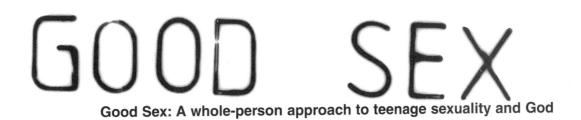

GOOD SEX

Good Sex: A whole-person approach to teenage sexuality and God

Jim Hancock and Kara Eckmann Powell

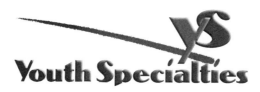

Youth Specialties

ZondervanPublishingHouse
Grand Rapids, Michigan

A Division of HarperCollinsPublishers

Good Sex: A whole-person approach to teenage sexuality & God

Copyright © 2001 by Jim Hancock and Kara Eckmann Powell

Youth Specialties Books, 300 S. Pierce St., El Cajon, CA 92020, are published by Zondervan Publishing House, 5300 Patterson, S.E., Grand Rapids, MI 49530.

Unless otherwise noted, all Scripture references are taken from the *Holy Bible: New International Version* (North American Edition), copyright © 1973, 1978, 1984 by the International Bible Society. Used by permission of Zondervan Bible Publishers.

Edited by Tamara Rice, Lorna McFarland Hartman, and Dave Urbanski
Additional contributions by James Prior
Cover design and photographs by Proxy
Interior design by Razdezignz

Printed in the United States of America

01 02 03 04 05 06 07 / / 10 9 8 7 6 5 4 3 2 1

To Susan, the woman of my dreams since 1972.
—J. H.

To my husband, Dave: your model of gentle strength
helps me be the woman I want to be.
—K. E. P.

read me

An essential primer for using Good Sex

Let's just get this out on the table: the biblical values around sex are counter-intuitive. Our culture, our bodies—every fiber of our beings—scream for sex early and often. And early and often is not exactly a biblical approach to responsible, intimate, disciplined, pleasurable, committed, passionate sex. So we're in a bit of a bind. Either our culture and our bodies are right about sexual fulfillment—and God just forgot to mention it was all a joke—or God is perfectly clear and correct about the sexual experiences that are most fulfilling, useful, helpful, and ultimately pleasurable, and we're just having a tough time understanding how to get there.

So it doesn't take a genius to see we're raising kids who feel emotionally and spiritually upside down regarding sex. And it's no secret that the church has lost its voice, partly from confusion and fear, partly from screaming itself hoarse. Those of us who aren't scared silent suffer a sort of cultural laryngitis—people see our lips moving but can't make out what we're saying.

Wouldn't it be nice to have reasonable, direct, honest, genuine, hopeful conversations about sex? Wouldn't it be good for our kids to hear us speak of God's good gifts in glowing, optimistic terms? Wouldn't it be wonderful to discuss sex without fear or anger or pretense?

We can, if we really want to. *Good Sex* is presented with that hope. Here are the big ideas behind ***Good Sex***:

- We're created in God's image, male and female.
- Sexuality is a wonderful, complex gift that takes a lifetime to explore.
- Sex touches every part of us: our bodies, of course, but also our minds, emotions, spirits, and every relationship we have—including our families and the God who made us.
- Sex is affected by our brokenness and wrongdoing, just like everything else about us.
- Sex can be rescued and renewed by the grace of Christ, just like everything else about us.

Good Sex helps kids look at sex in the broad context of their whole lives. More precisely, ***Good Sex*** helps *youth workers* help their students understand sex in the context of their whole lives.

If our *strategy* is to look at sex in the context of the whole person, our *tactics* involve a collection of self-contained-but-still-connected program elements—bite-sized experiences to get kids thinking and talking about God's gift of sex.

Good Sex is organized into seven chapters:

- **Sex Talk**—Helping kids respond to the cultural messages they're wading through—or maybe more accurately, swimming through
- **Sexual Identity**—Helping kids think about the forces that shape their sexuality
- **Intimacy**—Helping kids think about dating and nonsexual closeness
- **Desire**—Helping kids understand their appetites and needs
- **Boundaries**—Helping kids know what to do with their sexuality
- **Responsibility**—Helping kids take sexual responsibility
- **Do-Overs**—Helping kids experience mercy, repentance, forgiveness, and restoration

(We've also added **The Stuff at the Back of the Book**: Plumbing and Wiring—FAQs, Back-to-Basics Biology, and All the Sex in the Bible.)

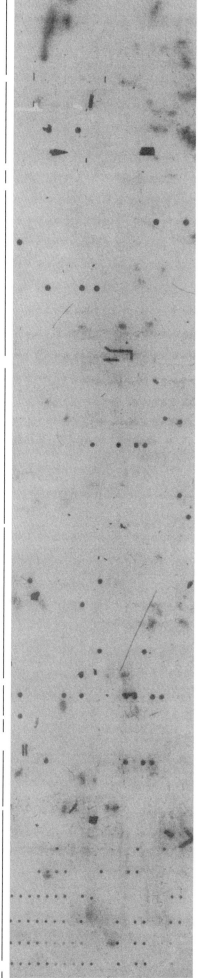

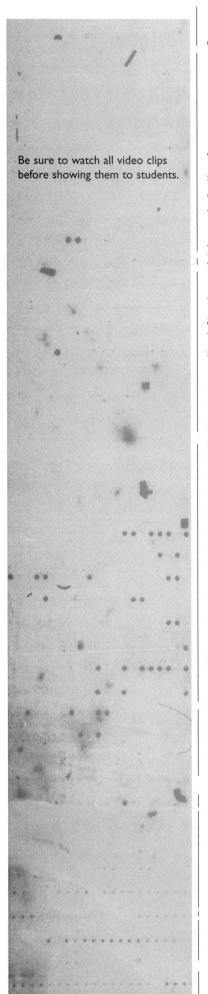

Be sure to watch all video clips before showing them to students.

Each chapter includes a lesson plan you can complete from beginning to end, comprising three elements:

- **In Our Own Words** is an opening group activity or discussion.
- **Word from God** is a Bible study.
- **The Last Word** is a concluding activity for personal reflection, sharing, and application.

This probably goes without saying but we want to be clear: your teaching style, how students respond to the discussion, and the degree to which you integrate the hand-outs—as well as the way you use them—will affect how much time each lesson takes. You're in control here.

The lesson is followed by **In Other Words**, a collection of additional activities you can use to extend your group learning or replace an element in the lesson plan with one you like better.

We've tried to make this organization clear enough so you can hand lessons to volunteers, give them about 20 minutes to prepare, and they can use them in small groups while you're off at a health spa (praying for your volunteers, of course). Yet we've also tried to make it flexible enough that you or another leader can prayerfully and intentionally customize it to your own setting.

There's logic to the order of the chapters, but the table of contents does *not* reflect a steadfast conviction about the order in which you should cover the material. **SexTalk** is a relatively low-risk place to start. It's at the beginning to give you a chance to assess what your group knows and thinks and how ready students are for some of the more challenging material. **Do-Overs** is significantly more challenging because it deals with brokenness. So it's at the end. But don't withhold the good news about God's restoration if you sense it ought to be included during any other session. (So it's a good idea to be familiar with **Do-Overs** *before* you start teaching any lesson.) If, from time to time during this process, you sense the need to proclaim mercy and forgiveness in Jesus, do it. Dip into the **Do-Overs** chapter for words of comfort and hope. Speak the truth about God's forgiveness to those who know they really need it.

Now for the program elements called **In Other Words**. You may be wondering, "Why create a bunch of extra resources that aren't part of a lesson plan? Why complicate things?" Glad you asked.

The simple answer is that we know youth groups, but we don't know *your* youth group. We don't know your theology, history, gifts, skills, or community, and (maybe most importantly) we don't know your boss. But what we do know is, the more experienced you are, the more likely it is you'll take whatever we do and rearrange it to fit your situation. You have to. We know that because that's what we've done with youth ministry resources for years. So we made it easy for you to customize *Good Sex*. If you see something in the lesson plan that doesn't bowl you over, replace it with something that does (as if you needed our permission).

And now for the more complicated answer:

In the real world, kids encounter sexual information and experiences in a process that stretches over decades. And out of that process—or in the middle of it—they construct their ideas and values about sex. And out of those ideas and values, they act. Most of that information—and quite a bit of the experience—is indirect. Kids read, listen, watch television and movies, hang out with friends and acquaintances. They watch their parents and other adults. They watch their siblings and peers. They experience sexual arousal (and it takes them by surprise).

From all these impressions, they construct a picture of what sex is—or what it appears to be. And from that picture come their sexual attitudes, opinions, and actions. The picture is updated as they encounter new information and experiences, and—even in adulthood—the picture is never complete as long as they're learning.

Contrast that with most teaching (distinct from learning) about sex. Most of what kids get directly from adults is much less a *process* and much more a *confrontation*: *"Here are the facts, remember them. These are the boundaries, don't cross them. This is the truth, believe it."*

If we agree that experience is the best teacher (not the preferred teacher, perhaps, but the most effective), which of these seems likely to be more influential: process or confrontation? We believe **Good Sex** should be more of a process than a confrontation because we believe that's how people—especially kids—learn best.

"But I've got to make my point!" you say.

Yes, you do. So why not make it with real energy and an effective feedback loop so you can find out which points you're actually making and how to finish what you started?

An ancient Hebrew liturgy celebrates a process of leading kids into loving obedience to their invisible Creator. This liturgy says, in part:

> Hear, O Israel: The Lord our God, the Lord is one. Love the Lord
> your God with all your heart and with all your soul and with all your
> strength. These commandments that I give you today are to be upon
> your hearts. Impress them on your children. Talk about them when
> you sit at home and when you walk along the road, when you lie
> down and when you get up. Tie them as symbols on your hands and
> bind them on your foreheads. Write them on the doorframes of your
> houses and on your gates. (Deuteronomy 6:4-9)

That's process. If you want to impress the next generation with biblical values around sex, it's the way we're recommending you do it, too. We don't believe an annual sex talk—or even the old six-week series—goes far enough to help kids wrestle with (and finally get pinned by) what the Bible says about sex. We believe the topic demands to be included in youth ministry as a subtext throughout the year—it's certainly a subtext in kids' lives, and they face new questions all the time. Here are a few ways we've tried to help you do that.

At the end of every lesson, you'll find reproducible handouts that help students personalize what they've learned from various activities and discussions. You can use these for further large-group discussion, for more intimate small-group conversations, or as tools for students' individual, personal reflection. (You can tell which activities come with handouts by looking in the nearby "You'll Need" box.)

We recommend you spread the activities from **In Other Words** across your year: ten minutes here, an evening there. Wherever it fits the larger process of youth ministry to the whole person. Once you start thinking about it, you'll probably see a host of topics that relate to sexuality: family relationships, emotions, school, temptation, peer pressure, media—the list goes on and on.

We created a book for kids called *What (Almost) Nobody Will Tell You about Sex*. It's a process-centered resource that invites kids to consider, understand, and surrender their sexuality to the God who loves them and made them sexual.

As you go through *What (Almost) Nobody Will Tell You about Sex*, you'll notice that while some elements run parallel to the Leader's Guide, the student book contains additional elements not found there. This is no accident. We view *What (Almost) Nobody Will Tell You about Sex* primarily as a tool that encourages students to process this material on their own—either outside the group or in smaller discussion groups within the larger gathering—so your kids can reflect upon their thoughts and feelings in deeper (perhaps more private) ways.

But if you want to use the Leader's Guide and *What (Almost) Nobody Will Tell You about Sex* in tandem during your meetings (and you can!), here's what we suggest: Be sure to familiarize yourself with the supplemental elements in the student book.

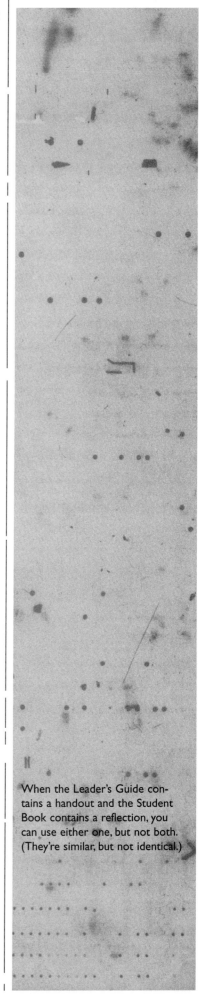

When the Leader's Guide contains a handout and the Student Book contains a reflection, you can use either one, but not both. (They're similar, but not identical.)

They're listed in the outer column near the end of each chapter (before the handouts). Whenever you think it's appropriate, encourage small group leaders to use these additional elements as discussion starters or follow-up questions, or encourage your students to go over a page on their own. For additional copies of *What (Almost) Nobody Will Tell You about Sex*, call 800-776-8008 or visit your Christian bookseller.

Be a participant as much as you can. When you're processing your own sexual experiences, you're better able to help kids in processing theirs. That's why we included "Reflect a Moment"—questions for *you* to think about—at the beginning of each chapter.

We've also included two additional resources:

• **Helping Parents with *Good Sex*** (page 15), on how to communicate effectively with your students' parents

• **Partnering with Your Youth Pastor** (page 16), a letter you can give to your senior pastor, CE director, or elder board to facilitate support for teaching *Good Sex*. It's a good idea to have the backing of church leadership before embarking on this topic.

Hands-On: Practical suggestions for leading a group through *Good Sex*

Make the group safe. Storytelling accomplishes something no other method can accomplish—it makes the group safe. Creating a safe group is critical, because people don't learn much when they have their guards up. Honest storytelling works because it meets the first requirement of the safe group: *Someone has to go first.*

Divide into same-sex groups. We suggest this to create a safe place for kids to discuss explosive sexual and gender issues. The vulnerability a teenager feels about the subject of sex will be respected—and the teenager will feel more encouraged to speak freely—when personal topics are discussed in a same-sex setting. It's possible to accidentally neutralize this safety by having a youth leader of the opposite sex leading the group.

Make room for silence. Silence may mean everybody's confused, asleep, mentally absent, or thinking. The only way to find out which one it is, is to ask. They'll usually tell you.

Make room for distraction. My peer leadership group was bouncing off the walls and I was irritated. I asked, "Is there something else we should be doing tonight?"

"No, sorry," somebody said. "It's just a weird day."

"Why weird?" I wanted to know.

"There was a suicide after school yesterday, and another last night. When the word got out this morning two more kids tried."

Oh.

I learned to ask this question whenever groups got squirrelly.

Trust Jesus with your group. Jesus was, after all, the master at leading groups.

Don't let deep water get you in hot water. Talking honestly about sex can create a sense of closeness in a group, and this can be arousing. Youth workers aroused by vulnerable kids are in a dangerous position. These issues of intimacy may also arise between fellow youth workers.

Learn to guard your heart and refrain from full frontal hugs. Always have potentially volatile conversations with students in public places or with an open office door.

Tell another adult where you're going *every* time you meet with a student and what kinds of issues you're dealing with (without breaking confidences).

Ask good questions. Anytime your group seems really *with* you on something you're teaching, ask variations on these three questions to find out what the kids' understanding is:

Q: What's the most significant thing you saw/heard/thought/felt? (This question gets at their perceptions.)

Q: Why do you suppose that seems so important to you? (This question gets at their intellectual and emotional response.)

Q: What do you think you might want to do about that? (This question gets at their intentions.)

Resources for Helping Kids with the Heavy Stuff

Good Sex can be "risky bidnez." If you make your room safe, there's always the chance some kid will admit or proclaim something shocking. So you'll have to decide right then and there to what degree you'll deal with whatever that kid said—and what should be reserved for a more private dialog after the meeting.

If kids reveal things about their sexual experiences that are troubling, frightening, even dangerous, don't freak out. Chances are if they choose to trust you with difficult stories about sexual abuse, they won't be going off the deep end anytime soon. They've probably carried the story silently for a while, and you've merely given them the impression that you can help. You can! You probably won't solve anything for them, but you can help them get the help they need. So, don't freak out. Take a deep breath, express your sympathy, and listen intently.

Chances are—and that's about 99 chances out of 100, so please assume this applies to you—you are what most states call a *mandated reporter*. That means if, after you hear a student's story, you believe that a reasonable person would call it sexual abuse, the law requires you to report it.

If you're not sure how to do that, use one or more of these resources:

• Begin with the senior staff member in your church or organization. That person will probably know what to do. But if you're convinced the situation is real and your staff leader seems confused or you fear he will sweep it under the rug, be sure to take other steps.

• Call the head counselor or vice principal at the student's school. Ask for help with understanding your legal responsibilities. See if that person will interview the student involved (with or without you present) and help you assess the seriousness of the situation. In the highly unlikely event the kid is lying, the school official will be a good backup. Chances are the official will be willing to call the sheriff, police, or child protective services (or whatever it's called where you live). Law enforcement jurisdictions can be confusing, and it's easy to get lost in the system. School personnel have probably already been through this, and they are likely to walk you through it, if you ask humbly.

• Get in touch with a trustworthy counselor or therapist and ask her to be a resource.

• If you go through all these channels and you believe nothing is happening, start again at the top, express your frustration and humbly ask for help. Be the widow in Luke 18 who keeps coming to the judge for justice until he pays attention.

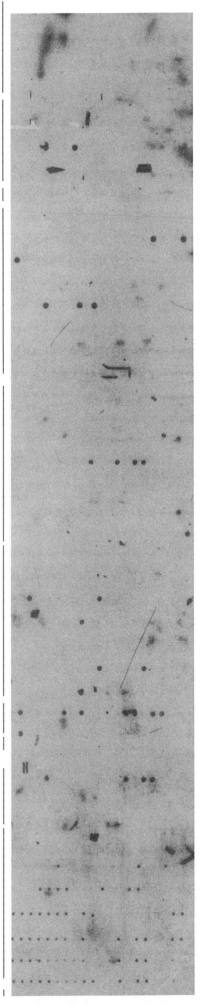

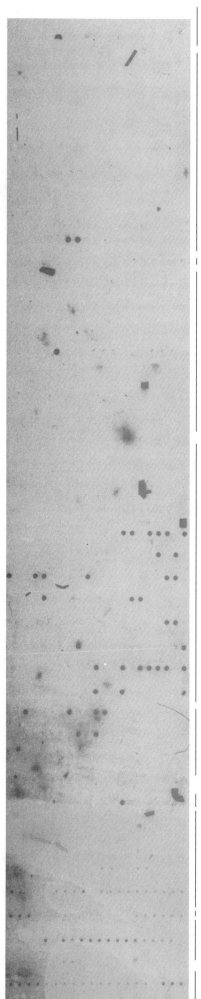

You're a poor youth worker looking for justice in a system where you probably don't feel at home. That's okay. Keep after it. If you don't give up, someone will listen to you eventually. But don't showboat. Don't parade around city hall or call press conferences to put people on the spot. You're most likely to get through the system by building relationships, not by tearing them down.

• Let your kids know about the Girls and Boys Town hotline: 800-448-3000. Girls and Boys Town offers a full range of help. Let kids know about this number for friends or for themselves. The hotline will send a stack of kid-friendly business cards if you ask nicely.

• The number for Childhelp USA is 800-4-A-CHILD. This organization specializes in sexual abuse assistance.

• If you fear for a kid's safety and can't seem to get the help you need locally, you can call 800-NEW-LIFE (New Life Treatment Centers' in-hospital psychiatric program) for recommendations on how to proceed. They won't try to sell you anything, and they'll give you the best information available.

Like we said earlier, using *Good Sex* is risky. The content is frank, honest, and challenging. And that demands that you model the behavior for your students. That can be scary—but even more so for your kids! So, as the walls and pretenses come crumbling down (hopefully), get ready to love and understand your students as you never have before.

Helping Parents with *Good Sex*

As you use *Good Sex,* here are three goals for communicating with parents to keep in mind:

1. Informing parents about the sexual pressures, thoughts, and feelings bombarding their students, and how kids are holding up under them.

2. Involving parents in their child's sex education, instead of abdicating it to the sex ed instructor at school—or to you!

3. Encouraging parents as they take steps, even baby steps, in discussing the all-too-often-taboo subject of sex with their own teens.

Here is a collection of ideas to help reach those goals.

- Forward information from each lesson to parents, especially any lists or provocative comments students make (keeping students anonymous, of course). Transcribe valuable tidbits and send them via email or through an old-fashioned letter.

- Send a prayer newsletter to parents to let them know what you're covering when—and how they can be praying. *Make schedule, utilize prayer ministry*

- Ahead of time, ask a parent you respect to be on call for an extended length of time—six to 12 months—to help other parents navigate through their students' tricky questions or struggles. *— Candy*

- Enlist a team of parents to contact the rest of the parents of your students to see what else your ministry can do to help.

- Send out encouraging, anonymous stories from students about how their parents have helped them deal with and understand sex.

- Host a parent seminar: "Talking with Your Teens about Sex." *— Candy, Nikki*

- Ask adults to share personal testimonies during your ~~youth group~~ *Sunday School* meetings about how they handled sex when they were teens.

- Organize a no-holds-barred parent panel on marriage and sexuality where kids get to anonymously ask the questions. *K to kids*

- Establish a parent advisory board to help all your parents with teen sex and other issues.

- Recommend to parents TV shows and magazines that reflect what their teens deal with sexually.

- Send copies of magazine articles (Christian or secular), as well as song lyrics, to parents to keep them informed on what their kids deal with sexually.

- Take a case study from each lesson and send it to parents with a few suggested discussion questions they could use with their own kids.

- Suggest that families hook up with other families to discuss these ideas. It might actually be easier for kids *and* parents to talk about sex with others around.

Parent meeting at end of curriculum

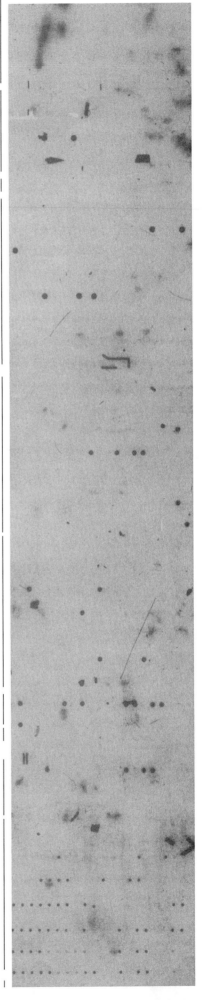

PARTNERING WITH YOUR YOUTH PASTOR

Teaching teens about sex is the youth pastor's job, right?

Well, partly.

Actually, as the youth worker's senior pastor or supervisor, your partnership is crucial to this curriculum's effectiveness in giving students a compass to navigate dangerous sexual waters. Here are some specific reasons your help is needed:

• Social science research consistently confirms the number-one influence in students' lives is not their friends, but their parents. Your position accords you a different level of influence than your youth pastor. You're likely to have more personal contact with parents, and greater authority (perhaps even greater credibility) because of your leadership.

• Parents are more likely to take the content of this series seriously if they know you and other church leaders are fully supportive.

• Some parents may have strong feelings about and reactions to what's being taught. Your youth pastor and adult volunteers need your prayer, advice, and support.

Here are some specific steps you can take to heighten the effectiveness of this series:

• Make sure your church has an explicit, written policy about reporting suspected child sexual abuse. If you're unsure what that policy should be, contact your denomination, a nearby church or school, or call your city or county child protective services office to get advice. If past or present sexual abuse is suspected, make sure you and the youth pastor are both clear on who should be contacted and what should be done.

• Help your youth pastor and adult volunteers identify affordable counselors and therapists who are Christians.

• Consider conducting a whole-church series on sexuality.

• Ask the adult classes and small groups connected with your church to focus some teaching, sharing, and accountability around sexuality.

• Host a marriage seminar so that parents can get the training and encouragement they need in all aspects of their relationship, including sex.

• Sponsor a parenting seminar to help parents know how to ask and respond to sensitive questions about their kids' sexuality.

This curriculum is designed to help your youth worker meet kids where they are, rather than where they're supposed to be (as you're painfully aware, we Christians are seldom where we're supposed to be). **Good Sex** invites students to embrace the biblical ideal of chastity until marriage.

We hope you'll do everything you can to encourage your youths as they consider how to be faithful stewards of God's great gift of sex.

before you teach this lesson...

Suppose you came to a country where you could fill a theatre by simply bringing a covered plate onto the stage and then slowly lifting the cover so as to let every one see, just before the lights went out, that it contained a mutton chop or a bit of bacon, would you not think that in that country something had gone wrong with the appetite for food?

—C. S. Lewis, *Mere Christianity* (Macmillan)

Something has gone wrong with our appetite for sex. By virtually any objective measure, our *cultural* preoccupation with sex has grown out of proportion to its actual significance. That may be hard to see since—other than more convenient access to pornography—not much has changed in the last decade.

Nothing has changed for the *kids* we serve. They've grown up largely unprotected from what grownups cynically refer to as *adult content*. Our younger brothers and sisters never knew a world without home video and cable sex, descriptive sexual language on pop radio, one-click access to Internet material that might have gotten their grandfathers kicked out of the house—or maybe even thrown in jail.

They also never knew a world without HIV/AIDS and rampant outbreaks of sexually transmitted infections—a world where careless sex can sterilize or even kill.

Telling kids how much things have changed doesn't make sense. It's like telling a porpoise the ocean used to be a nicer place to live. There's not much he can do with that information, is there?

So what do we tell our students? How do we equip them for life in the world where they live instead of in some Neverland where children don't wrestle with sexuality? Do we throw up our hands or dig in our heels? Do we ignore biblical messages written "too long ago and too far away" to be much use in the 21st century? Alter them to fit modern sensibilities? Or hunker down and defend our tiny square of turf until the last of us dies off and the world goes to hell?

Oddly enough, what the Bible says about sex may be more helpful than ever. Most everybody agrees we're in a mess. We're sexually confused and nobody seems to be doing much to clear things up. But almost no one wants to go back to pretending people don't think about sex until their wedding night. No one looks at the previous era of sneaky sex and thinks people were nobler because they lied about their behavior. And who in his right mind wants to go back into hiding about sexual abuse, leaving women and children vulnerable to assault?

This is no commendation for where we are now. Things are messy. But not messier than what's recorded in the Bible. People think the Bible is hopelessly naïve about modern sex. It's not. The Bible's message flourished in places where the sexual norms were far more abusive than modern western culture. Those folks lived in places where male and female prostitution was part of religious life—so just imagine life among the irreligious! They lived in towns where sacrificing girls was the main event at the shrine up on the hill. They lived in cities where boys were sex objects for wealthy men. They lived in cultures where women were property—collected, traded, used, and discarded. And no one raised an eyebrow, let alone a helping hand.

The people of God blew into those cultures like a fresh, but very strange, breeze. They brought hope and a wind of change. And not so much by their words as by their lives.

God's people reinvented the family by introducing committed marriage, instilling respect for women, and protecting and nurturing children instead of exploiting them.

Culture is the language, economy, spirituality, media, work, play, and social relationships that shape your environment.

These ideas were huge, not because smart people wrote about them, but because ordinary people lived them out. Think of what we know about sexual abuse—most abusers were themselves victims of abuse when they were young. There's every reason to believe it's always been that way. Which means that adult believers who were abused as children chose to break the cycle of abuse—they chose to give better than they got. Adult believers chose to treat their wives as partners instead of property. Adult believers who grew up one way chose another way to live by the power of God's Spirit, so children weren't disposable, marriages weren't temporary, and sex wasn't violent. That was world-changing stuff.

Maybe it's time to do that again. Somehow, the church has lost the thread of sexual wholeness. We still talk a good game, but people don't listen anymore.

So maybe it's time to stop talking and instead, steadily but quietly, help kids grow into their sexuality healthy and whole. We can do that with God's grace, not because we're good, but because God is so very good. Maybe it's time for adult believers to give better than we got. It's within our reach.

what's in this lesson...

IN OUR OWN WORDS	**LOVELINE** your students' reactions to MTV's "Loveline" scenarios
	NOTHING BUT THE TRUTH...MAYBE video discussion starter about the sources of sexual messages
WORD FROM GOD	**TO OBEY OR NOT TO OBEY** a look at Genesis 2 and 3
THE LAST WORD	**BOMBARDMENT** a discussion starter about absorbing God's views on sex
	WHERE IN THE WORLD ARE YOU? an anonymous survey to gauge where your students are at
IN OTHER WORDS	See page 23 for additional teaching activities

reflect a moment...

To help your students most effectively, you need to make every effort to process your own sexual experiences, questions, and struggles. Here are some questions to get you thinking:

Q: If a totally objective stranger had absolute access to your life, where do you think she would say you got your ideas about sex?
- What influences do you think she would say were healthy for you?
- What influences do you think she would say were unhealthy?

Q: Forget about the totally objective stranger. What do you wish you had learned sooner?
- Is there anything you wish you could go back and unlearn?

Q: If you had just one hour to talk with kids about sex, what would you try to communicate?
- Why do you think that's so important?
- How would you try to communicate during that hour?

In our own ~~words~~

The types of questions and answers about sex that are tossed around in our culture.

How many of you have heard of the show "Loveline"? It airs nearly every night on the radio and is shown regularly on MTV. As I'm sure some of you are more than aware, this show consists of people calling up and asking Dr. Drew, Adam Carolla, and various special guests questions about their sexuality.

Here is just a sampling of actual questions asked during one of their shows.

Adam, 18 years old, calls in and says that when he was 16 he slept with his high school English teacher about 10 times. She got pregnant not long after and refused to have any more contact with him. He saw the baby recently and says that it looks exactly like him. He's sure the baby is his, but he doesn't know what to do.

Q: What advice do you think the "Loveline" hosts gave to Adam? Why do you think that?

Q: What advice do you think your youth leader would give to Adam? Why do you think that?

Q: What advice do you think Jesus would give Adam? Why do you think that?

The "Loveline" hosts told Adam to stay out of the situation because he has absolutely nothing to offer this child. It's better if the child never knows who his father is.

Toni, a 25-year-old female transvestite, calls in to ask for some advice. She slept with a girlfriend's fiancé. The girlfriend has no idea that her future marriage partner is thinking about becoming a transvestite as well. Should Toni tell her girlfriend what she knows?

Q: What advice do you think the "Loveline" hosts gave to Toni? Why do you think that?

Q: What advice do you think your youth leader would give to Toni? Why do you think that?

Q: What advice do you think Jesus would give Toni? Why do you think that?

The "Loveline" hosts told Toni to stay out of it. Let them work this stuff out themselves.

Melissa, 19, was at a house with three male friends when they spiked her drink with speedball (part heroin, part cocaine). When she had completely lost control of her senses, these three so-called friends gang-raped her. That was six months ago. Since then, Melissa has had compulsive sex with over 30 men—all one-night stands. She doesn't know why she is doing this.

Q: What advice do you think the "Loveline" hosts gave to Melissa? Why do you think that?

Q: What advice do you think your youth leader would give to Melissa? Why do you think that?

If "Loveline" becomes irrelevant or goes away before you use this lesson, just change everything to the past tense. "There used to be a show called 'Loveline'..."

All questions were taken from the "Loveline" episode aired on July 25, 2000, on MTV.

In February 1999, the Henry J. Kaiser Family Foundation released a study indicating that two-thirds of prime time TV shows and 56 percent of all TV shows include sexual content. The shows with the most sex are soap operas, movies, and talk shows. According to this study, relatively few of these shows offer "responsible" sexual messages about contraceptive use, abstinence, or protection from sexually transmitted infections.

These findings prompted Health and Human Services secretary Donna E. Shalala to compare TV sex to the distorted mirror at a carnival fun house.

—*Cheryl Wetzstein,*
Washington Times (September 13, 1999)

YOU'LL NEED
- VCR or DVD player
- TV or video projection unit
- *Good Sex* video, cued to **"Nothing but the Truth"** [2:35]
- copies of **Nothing but the Truth...Maybe** (page 27), one per student
- pencils

Q: What advice do you think Jesus would give Melissa? Why do you think that?

The "Loveline" hosts told Melissa that she had a compulsive addiction to sex that had been triggered by this event. She was told to get counseling and hook up with an AA-type group.

Q: Given the advice that the "Loveline" hosts gave, would you recommend that a friend who is struggling with a sexual issue call in to try to talk to them? Why or why not?

At times, the hosts and guests of "Loveline" give straightforward and sympathetic advice. Granted, it's generally not based on anything related to God, but sometimes it still seems relevant.

But at other times, the advice of "Loveline" is less than healthy. I wonder if folks, even Christian folks, turn to places like "Loveline" because they believe that most churches and Christians are too scared to talk about sex in as real and honest a way as they do on "Loveline."

Q. Do you agree that most churches and Christians are scared to talk about sex in real and honest ways? Why or why not?

Q. How would you rate the quality of information you've received about sex from the church or from the Bible?
- From your friends?
- From TV and movies?
- From magazines?
- From the Internet?

Q. Where has the best and most helpful sexual info come from? Why do you think that is?

---

video discussion starter

NOTHING BUT THE TRUTH...MAYBE
VIDEO

Evaluating the quantity and quality of the sources of sexual messages we're exposed to.

Introduce and show the video clip. It portrays a variety of teens explaining how they've heard and learned about sex.

Q: What sources of sexual messages were mentioned in the video? What others can you think of that weren't mentioned in the video?
- Of these, what do you think are the most common sources of sexual information for teens?

Q: There seemed to be a common belief that sex ed at school wasn't very helpful. What do you think about that?

Q: Is it true that students get clean info from their parents but the dirty version from other kids at school? How would you even define clean, and how is it different from the dirty version?

Q: How comfortable do you think parents are talking to their own kids about sex? How comfortable do you think kids are talking to their parents about it?

Q: Many people would say that the sexual messages implied in the Bible are not positive. In fact, many would say that the Bible gives a very negative view of sexuality. Discuss this observation and give some reasons why people might think this.

Q: How does our youth group do in providing a place where positive and helpful sexual messages are given?

At this point, you might want to use the provocative and probing questions included in **Nothing but the Truth...Maybe** (page 27) as the basis for a deeper group discussion, as material to be covered in smaller group discussions, or as a tool for students to engage in individual, personal reflection.

word from God

Bible study

TO OBEY OR NOT TO OBEY

The link between sin and an unhealthy view of sexuality.

Let's have a look in Genesis to see where some of these distorted views of sexuality might have begun.

Read Genesis 2:18-25 with your students.

There was a time when there was no negative understanding of sexuality. God made Adam and Eve in his exact image and gave them the ability to be sexually active. This passage says that Adam and Eve had no shame about being naked.

Q: Why do you think Adam and Eve felt no shame about being naked?

Q: Do you agree there's a link between Adam and Eve having no shame about being naked and them having a healthy understanding of their own sexuality? Discuss this.

Q: Do you think it was God's ultimate design that there be nothing negative about sex between a man and a woman? Talk about this idea.

Ask a student volunteer to read what happened next in paradise from Genesis 3:1-8.

Q: After Adam and Eve disobeyed God's one and only commandment, why do you think the first thing they did was realize they were naked and cover themselves up?

Q: How do you think this first act of disobedience relates to all of the negative sexual messages and implications that we face today?

It seems that something big happened way back in the garden. A huge change developed in the way Adam and Eve viewed their bodies—and most likely their sexuality—before and after they disobeyed God. It also seems that many of the negative messages we face today come from the same type of rebellion and poor choices.

Q: Do you think that it's possible for us to regain a pure and beautiful understanding of sex? Why or why not?

Q: Do you think God still has a positive outlook on sexuality, or has sin made his view of sex more negative also?

For additional reflection and discussion on the link between disobedience and sexuality, use the questions from **To Obey or Not to Obey** (page 28 in this book) in large or small group discussions or as a tool for students' individual reflection.

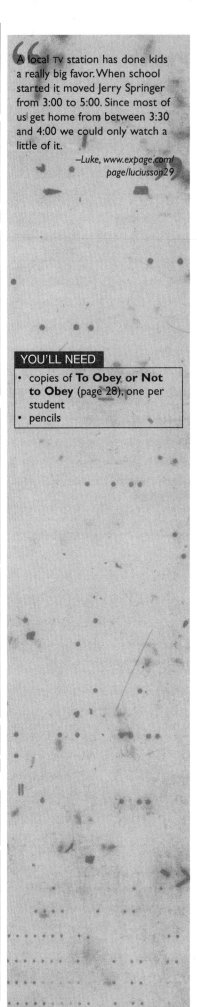

" A local TV station has done kids a really big favor. When school started it moved Jerry Springer from 3:00 to 5:00. Since most of us get home from between 3:30 and 4:00 we could only watch a little of it.

—Luke, www.expage.com/
page/luciusson29

YOU'LL NEED

- copies of **To Obey or Not to Obey** (page 28), one per student
- pencils

the last word

BOMBARDMENT

How to soak in more of God's messages about sex.

Read the following quote aloud.

> **A recent study concluded that an average American teen watches 14,000 sexual encounters a year on television alone. Most adolescents spend one second learning the discipline of intimacy for every hundred hours they absorb distorted images of intimacy from media and other kids.**
>
> **A movie like *Pretty Woman* is a wonderful case in point. Here is a very entertaining Hollywood film, which is purportedly about love. In fact it's only about the first stage of love, the romance of the mating ritual. Once the couple has mated, the movie ends. It is like 99 percent of the movies, stories, and books we read. Love, in this unreal model, is too easy, not a discipline but a series of conversations and little tiffs that lead to sex and marriage.**
>
> **To an adult who knows better, *Pretty Woman* is just good entertainment. To a boy, *Pretty Woman* teaches not discipline, but fantasy.**
> **—Michael Gurian, *The Wonder of Boys* (Tarcher/Putnam)**

Q: Do you think it's possible to live our lives so the sexual messages we don't consider helpful have little or no impact on our understanding of sexuality?

Q: Romans 12:2 says we should no longer be conformed to the pattern of this world but that we should be transformed by the renewing of our minds. What does this mean? How is this relevant to what we're talking about?

Q: Instead of the animal sacrifices described in the Old Testament, Paul invites all believers to be living sacrifices in verse 1. What do you think it means to be a *living sacrifice*? How would this affect what kinds of sexual messages we expose ourselves to?

Q: What are some things we can do to continually keep ourselves open to God's positive message of sexuality and block out the world's negative messages?

Absorbing more of God's views about sexuality than the distorted ones that surround us is no easy thing. Hard-core porn is just a mouse click away, and soft-core porn is on our cable stations every night. Many movies make it seem like it's socially acceptable to be sexually active early in your teenage years. This is without doubt one of the hardest things you will have to face in the Christian life. But it's possible to get a positive understanding of sexuality that's not repressive or binding. It comes from having a right relationship with God—the one who created sex in the first place.

WHERE IN THE WORLD ARE YOU?

Where we stand and where we want to go.

Hopefully this group can be a safe place for us to discuss the messages and pressures that are bombarding us about our sexuality. And hopefully we won't just stop there, but we'll figure out what God says to us both through the Bible and through each other. We don't want to waste anybody's time here—not yours or mine. To

---

When the Leader's Guide contains a handout and the Student Book contains a reflection, you can use either one, but not both. (They're similar, but not identical.)

If your students are using *What (Almost) Nobody Will Tell You about Sex,* you can direct them to **Where in the World Are You?** (page 13).

YOU'LL NEED

- copies of **Where in the World Are You?** (page 29), one per student
- pencils

make sure we all understand the most important questions and issues we're facing, I'd like to give you time to complete **Where in the World Are You?** (page 29) and give it back to me. I'm not going to do handwriting analysis or anything on it to try to figure out who wrote what. It's completely anonymous, so hopefully you'll feel free to identify where you're at right now, as well as where you'd like to be in the future.

After students complete their handouts, if you have time, divide into smaller groups and have students share one or two things they wrote. Make sure to collect all surveys so that you can compile the results and use them to guide your use of everything else in this kit.

In other words

active evaluation
WHERE DID YOU LEARN ABOUT SEX?

The sources that give us the most reliable information about sex—other than youth workers, who are obviously the most reliable sources.

Tape the paper signs across the front of your room in a continuum beginning with LIES and ending with TOTALLY TRUE. Read the following sources of sexual messages one at a time and ask students to identify what they have learned about sex from each and how true-to-life that information is. After you've discussed an item, have a student write it down on a sheet of paper and tape it to the sign that matches the majority of your group's opinion about its accuracy.

- romance novels
- music
- sex ed
- soap operas
- movies
- visual porn
- locker room swagger
- sleepover gossip and confessionals
- parent-child sex talks
- youth group talks
- Christian books and speakers
- other

Q: Why do you think some sources are more reliable than others?
- How do you judge the reliability of a source?
- Do you think there's any difference in the reliability of sources for boys and girls? Why?

Q: If someone came to you for advice on where to go to learn about sex, where would you send that person? Why?

For additional personal and reflective questions about the sources of sexual messages, turn to **Where Did You Learn about Sex?** (page 31 in this book) and use the questions for large or small group discussion, or as a handout for students' individual reflection.

voting game
IN THE BIBLE/NOT IN THE BIBLE

God expects us to be passionate about romance and sex—ain't that good news?!

There are two ways to do this exercise—you choose.
   The first is to get two pieces of cardboard and write IN THE BIBLE on one, NOT IN THE BIBLE on the other. Tape these signs up on the two opposite sides or walls of your meeting room. As you read the following passages out loud—some of which are in

This activity has been designed for you to gauge where in the world your group is when it comes to sexual matters. Emphasize that this is an *anonymous* activity you'll use to gauge what will and won't work as you go through *Good Sex.*

If your students are using *What (Almost) Nobody Will Tell You about Sex,* you can direct them to **Where Did You Learn about Sex?** (page 11).

YOU'LL NEED
- copies of **Where Did You Learn about Sex?** (page 31) one per student
- pencils
- paper signs, each of which says one of the following:
   LIES
   STUPID
   NONSENSE
   NICE TRY
   WARMER
   HOT
   TOTALLY TRUE
- sheets of paper
- tape
- broad-tip marker

I wish someone had told me about the mechanical parts that just aren't very sexy at all; just the mechanics of making everything fit right.
   —Brian, on being prepared for his wedding night

YOU'LL NEED
- two pieces of paper or cardboard large enough to write NOT IN THE BIBLE and IN THE BIBLE so that students can see it from wherever they're sitting
- copies of **In the Bible/Not in the Bible** (page 32), one per student
- pencils
- broad-tip marker

the Bible and some of which are not—have your students move to either side of the room depending on whether they think that passage is in the Bible or not. Whichever student arrives last at either of the two sides of the room has to tell the whole group why he does or doesn't think that passage is in the Bible.

The second way is to just read the following passages out loud, one at a time, and get your students to corporately vote for whether they think it's in the Bible or not in the Bible.

Have fun as you read these passages, emphasizing their romance with your tone of voice and facial expressions. (By the way, all the biblical quotes are from the Song of Songs, and all the nonbiblical love lines are from Margaret Browning's *Poems of Love* [St. Martin's Press]).

> Let him kiss me with the kisses of his mouth—for your love is more delightful than wine. (Song of Songs 1:2)
>
> How handsome you are, my lover! Oh, how charming! (Song of Songs 1:16)
>
> Breathless, we flung us on the windy hills, laughed in the sun, and kissed the lovely grass. (*Poems of Love*)
>
> My lover is mine and I am his; he browses among the lilies. (Song of Songs 2:16)
>
> You and I have met but for an instant...But the eyes, voice audible—the soul's lips, stirred the depths of thought and feeling in me. (*Poems of Love*)
>
> She drips herself with water, and her shoulders glisten as silver. (*Poems of Love*)
>
> Your two breasts are like two fawns, like twin fawns of a gazelle that browse among the lilies. (Song of Songs 4:5)
>
> We made the universe to be our home, our nostrils took the wind to be our breath, our hearts are massive towers of delight. (*Poems of Love*)
>
> You have stolen my heart, my sister, my bride; you have stolen my heart with one glance of your eyes. (Song of Songs 4:9)
>
> I belong to my lover, and his desire is for me. (Song of Songs 7:10)

The Bible is not silent about important issues like sex, love, romance, and dating. Some people like to gloss over these passages in the Bible and pretend they aren't there. The truth is that God is really concerned about giving us positive sexual messages. Unfortunately for us, though, his positive words about sex get drowned out by all the negative and flat-out wrong sexual messages that flood over us.

To help students work through the clash between what many believe God thinks about human sexuality and what he actually says, distribute copies of **In the Bible/Not in the Bible** (page 32 in this book) and use its contents for your large group discussion, smaller group discussions, or as a tool for students' individual, personal reflections.

IF NOT HERE, THEN WHERE?

YOU'LL NEED

- five large sheets of butcher paper—on each one, write one of these words or phrases:
    1. WHAT SEX IS
    2. EMBARRASSED
    3. AFRAID
    4. IGNORANT
    5. WHAT SEX ISN'T
- paper
- masking tape,
- broad-tip marker
- copies of **If Not Here, Then Where?** (page 33), one per student
- pencils

Making our group the kind of place where sex can be discussed openly and safely.

The five phrases or words you posted around the room will serve as a scale to help students evaluate their various sources of sexual information.

Post the signs in the order listed along a wall or around the room to serve as a scale to help students evaluate their various sources of sexual information.

Q: What are some sources that give you information about sex?

As students give their ideas, write each idea on a separate sheet of paper. Ideas may include movies, Internet, magazine articles, magazine ads, siblings, radio, TV shows, TV ads, parents, church, locker room gossip, friends, teachers, school counselors, cousins, or overhearing others.

Q: Let's vote on where each of these sources belongs on the continuum between WHAT SEX IS and WHAT SEX ISN'T. In general where do you think movies go? (And so on.)

As you call out the source on each sheet of paper, tape it near the sign the group votes for. You may want two or three assistants to help with the postings.

Q: Are there any sheets at WHAT SEX IS?
- What makes these sources of information seem like a place where you can get the whole truth and nothing but the truth?

Q: Are there any sheets at WHAT SEX ISN'T?
- What makes these sources of information seem so unreliable?

Q: Where do you think our youth group belongs up here?
- What is it about our group that makes it fit that spot on the scale?
- What kind of students would make our group a safe place to talk about the reality of sex?
- What would we have to change to become that kind of group?

Talk with your group about confidentiality using ideas like these.

> **Let's talk about confidentiality. Here's the standard I'm going to ask you to consider.**
>
> - **Unless someone's life appears to be in immediate danger, what we say here stays here when we leave here—no repeating, no gossip, no "prayer requests" to others outside the group. Does that seem fair? If it does, I'd like each of us to say something like this right out loud—I'll go first: "I'm willing to keep what we say here confidential unless someone's life is in danger, and I'm asking you to do the same thing."**
>
> - **If you believe someone's life is in immediate danger, here's what I'd like you to do:**
>
> - **First, please tell me and no one else.**
>
> - **If you can't track me down, please tell one of the other adults in the group and no one else.**

If your students are using *What (Almost) Nobody Will Tell You about Sex*, you can direct them to these additional pages: **Girls, Guys, and Changing Bodies; Pick One; Sexual Sanctuary** (pages 14, 16, 20).

• **If you can't track down another adult from the group, please tell our pastor, your school counselor, or your assistant principal, and no one else.**

• **When you finally track me down, even if you've told someone else, please tell me so I can follow up on it.**

The point is to protect each other's privacy, except when someone's life is in danger. Does that seem fair? If it doesn't, let's talk about it until we find something that does seem fair.

To conclude this activity, distribute copies of **If Not Here, Then Where?** (page 33 in this book), one per student, and ask them the questions in a large-group forum or smaller groups, or give them time to reflect and write their responses individually.

When they're all finished responding to these questions, invite students who feel prompted to change something about themselves with the hope of influencing the tone of the youth group to share that aloud in one or two sentences. You and your adult leaders might want to set the tone by sharing something you know you need to change, such as a fear that students will reject you if you share about your struggles or the false belief that in order to lead you have to be totally together and perfect.

Close in prayer, thanking God that he doesn't want you or any of his children to be static but he's always giving you opportunities to grow and deepen your relationship with him and with others in your community or youth group.

NOTHING BUT THE TRUTH...MAYBE

Reflect on these questions with your group or by yourself.

Q: Where do you get your most important information about sex?
- Why there?

Q: What do you think is the most important thing you've learned about sex so far?
- Why do you think that's so important?
- What effect would you say that information has on your behavior?

Q: What's the most useless thing you've learned about sex?
- Why do you consider that worthless?

Q: Do you think there's anywhere you can go to escape false messages about sex?

Q: What would you like to understand better about sex? Why?

TO OBEY OR NOT TO OBEY

Read Genesis 3:1-24

and then reflect on these questions.

Q: What's an early memory of consciously disobeying God where God said don't do this and you decided to do it anyway, or God said do this and you decided not to do it anyway? Reflect on what happened. Don't strain your brain—just think back a bit.
- When you finally came around and realized that you were being a banana head, do you recall wanting to make excuses like the woman in this story?
- Do you recall wanting to blame someone like the man in this story?
- What was the outcome of that disobedience? Is that different from more recent experiences?

Q: If you're like many people, you didn't learn your lesson in one step. How are you tempted to resist God these days?
- How do you think your resistance to God relates to your sexuality?
- Do you make excuses for disobeying God? If so, what are they?

Q: Can you identify any lasting effects from your disobedience to God in general? How about in your sexuality? Reflect on that.

Q: Genesis 3:21 describes God's care for the man and the woman in a single line, saying he "made garments of skin for Adam and his wife and clothed them." God looked out for them in spite of their disobedience. How have you seen God's care for you in spite of your resistance?

WHERE IN THE WORLD ARE YOU?

When it comes to our experience, our knowledge, and our awareness of friendship, dating, and romance, we're probably all over the map. Circle the percentage that indicates how much you agree with each statement if your youth group is discussing friendship, dating, and romance.

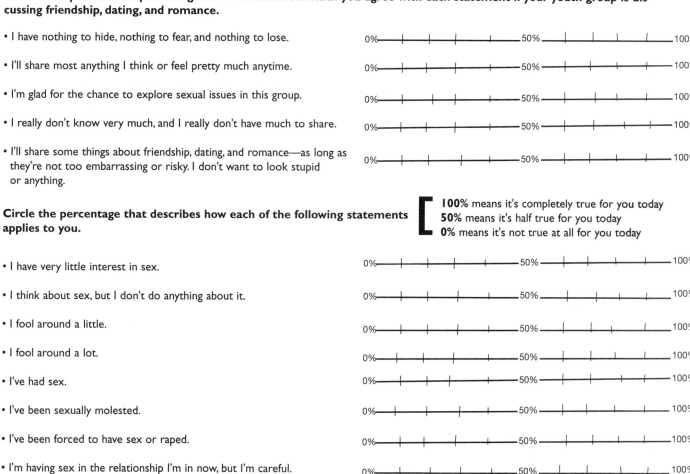

• I have nothing to hide, nothing to fear, and nothing to lose.

0%————————50%————————100%

• I'll share most anything I think or feel pretty much anytime.

0%————————50%————————100%

• I'm glad for the chance to explore sexual issues in this group.

0%————————50%————————100%

• I really don't know very much, and I really don't have much to share.

0%————————50%————————100%

• I'll share some things about friendship, dating, and romance—as long as they're not too embarrassing or risky. I don't want to look stupid or anything.

0%————————50%————————100%

Circle the percentage that describes how each of the following statements applies to you.

100% means it's completely true for you today
50% means it's half true for you today
0% means it's not true at all for you today

• I have very little interest in sex.

0%————————50%————————100%

• I think about sex, but I don't do anything about it.

0%————————50%————————100%

• I fool around a little.

0%————————50%————————100%

• I fool around a lot.

0%————————50%————————100%

• I've had sex.

0%————————50%————————100%

• I've been sexually molested.

0%————————50%————————100%

• I've been forced to have sex or raped.

0%————————50%————————100%

• I'm having sex in the relationship I'm in now, but I'm careful.

0%————————50%————————100%

• I've been having sex for a while and with a number of partners. I'm always very careful.

0%————————50%————————100%

• I used to have sex more than I do now.

0%————————50%————————100%

• I'm not sexually active right now, but that could change if the right person came along.

0%————————50%————————100%

• I've been tested for sexually transmitted infectionss since the last time I had sex.

0%————————50%————————100%

The last time I had sex was—

☐ in the last week
☐ in the last month
☐ in the last three months
☐ in the last six months
☐ in the last year
☐ in the last two years
☐ in the last three years
☐ more than three years ago
☐ never

"There came a moment about a year before my stroke in 1985 when I felt that pursuing multipartner sex was kind of pointless and pathetic.
—*Hugh Hefner, Playboy founder,*
(Details, April 1993)"

 (continued)

If we were going to talk about sexual issues in the group, circle the percentage that describes your interest level.

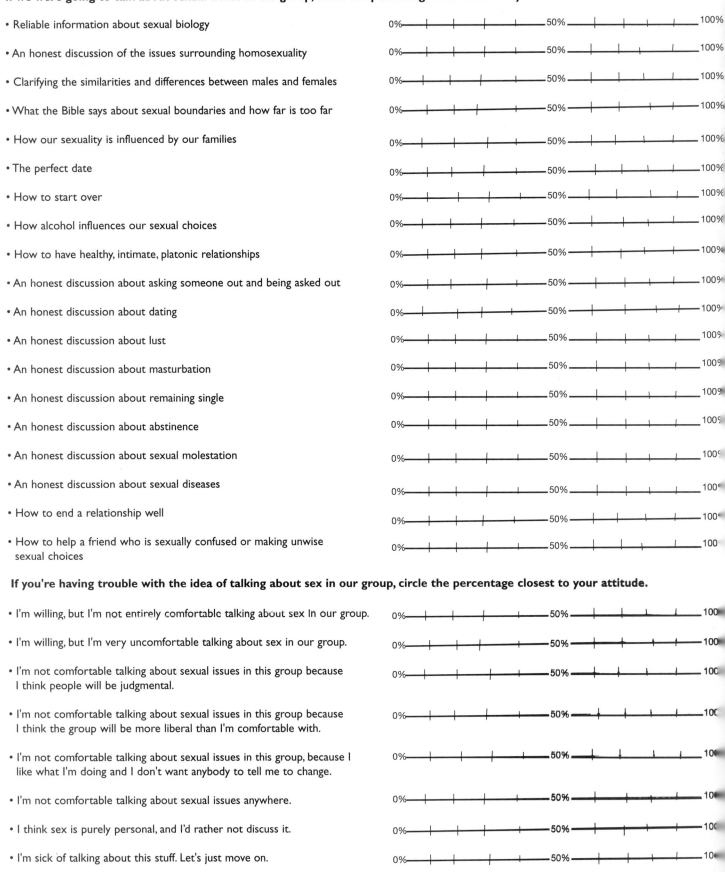

- Reliable information about sexual biology   0%————50%————100%
- An honest discussion of the issues surrounding homosexuality   0%————50%————100%
- Clarifying the similarities and differences between males and females   0%————50%————100%
- What the Bible says about sexual boundaries and how far is too far   0%————50%————100%
- How our sexuality is influenced by our families   0%————50%————100%
- The perfect date   0%————50%————100%
- How to start over   0%————50%————100%
- How alcohol influences our sexual choices   0%————50%————100%
- How to have healthy, intimate, platonic relationships   0%————50%————100%
- An honest discussion about asking someone out and being asked out   0%————50%————100%
- An honest discussion about dating   0%————50%————100%
- An honest discussion about lust   0%————50%————100%
- An honest discussion about masturbation   0%————50%————100%
- An honest discussion about remaining single   0%————50%————100%
- An honest discussion about abstinence   0%————50%————100%
- An honest discussion about sexual molestation   0%————50%————100%
- An honest discussion about sexual diseases   0%————50%————100%
- How to end a relationship well   0%————50%————100%
- How to help a friend who is sexually confused or making unwise sexual choices   0%————50%————100%

If you're having trouble with the idea of talking about sex in our group, circle the percentage closest to your attitude.

- I'm willing, but I'm not entirely comfortable talking about sex in our group.   0%————50%————100%
- I'm willing, but I'm very uncomfortable talking about sex in our group.   0%————50%————100%
- I'm not comfortable talking about sexual issues in this group because I think people will be judgmental.   0%————50%————100%
- I'm not comfortable talking about sexual issues in this group because I think the group will be more liberal than I'm comfortable with.   0%————50%————100%
- I'm not comfortable talking about sexual issues in this group, because I like what I'm doing and I don't want anybody to tell me to change.   0%————50%————100%
- I'm not comfortable talking about sexual issues anywhere.   0%————50%————100%
- I think sex is purely personal, and I'd rather not discuss it.   0%————50%————100%
- I'm sick of talking about this stuff. Let's just move on.   0%————50%————100%
- If you insist on talking about sex, let me know when you're done—I'll consider coming back to the group at that point.   0%————50%————100%

WHERE DID YOU LEARN ABOUT SEX?

Reflect on the following questions.

Q: So where have you been learning about sex?
- How reliable does that information seem to be so far?
- Where do you wish you had learned about sex?

Q: Are you surprised at the quality of information you've gotten from one source or another? Why is that?

Q: Have you gotten hurt by any bad information? If so, what was the source of the bad information?
- What happened?
- How did you feel about that?
- How did you work it out?
- Did you have anyone to help you process that?

Q: Is there any source you consider so poor you simply won't go there? Why is that?
- Is there any source so consistently helpful you would recommend it to someone who needs help?
- If so, what makes it so valuable to you?

Q: What other sources or people do you think would be reliable, but you haven't sought out yet? When do you think you could seek them out?

IN THE BIBLE/NOT IN THE BIBLE

Reflect on the following questions.

Q: Three words I would have used when we started this discussion to describe how I think God views romance and love would be—

1._____because—

2._____because—

3._____because—

Q: Given what I've just heard from the Song of Songs, three words that describe how God views romance and love would be—

1._____because—

2._____because—

3._____because—

Q: I feel like—

☐ Of course God cares about my dating relationships, because—

☐ I'm not clear where God stands, because—   ☐ I don't think God cares, because—

Q: If I viewed my dating relationships the way God did, the differences would be—

Q: Someone who I think understands God's view on romance and sexuality (and who I could talk to in the future) is—

IF NOT HERE, THEN WHERE? WHERE?

Q: What words describe how you feel about talking about sex in our youth group?
- What words do you wish described how you feel about discussing sex here?
- If there's a difference, reflect on that.

Q: What would you have to change to be the kind of person who could make our youth ministry a safe place to talk about the reality of sex?
- What do you have to lose by making that change?
- What could you gain?
- How do you think that change might influence our youth group?

Q: If you think there's no way you could talk about sex honestly in our group, is there an adult Christian who seems safe to talk to that you could approach?
- What would keep you from doing this?
- What would help you?

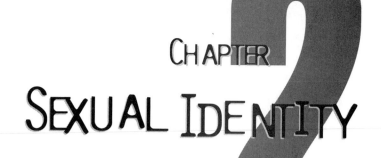

before you teach this lesson...

The first pages of the first book of the Bible say God made humans male and female: a matched set. Both are necessary for reproduction; each benefits from the unique-ness of the other. We're speaking in general here—your mileage may vary depending on the quality of men and women you know. Anyway, that's *sex*, that's *gender*. Two X chromosomes deliver a female, an X and a Y produce a male.

Sexual identity is a different matter. Sexual identity is how we experience our sex-uality, and what we think and how we feel about it. This has a lot to do with hor-mones—testosterone in boys and progesterone in girls. But it also has something to do with how we're treated by our families, friends, schools, mass media...the whole culture. That's what this chapter is mainly about.

From the day they're born, how children think about their sexuality is influenced by their families, friends, and communities. Women and men tell boys and girls how to act; children watch and learn from adults how it's really done. And they read, listen to the radio, go to the playground, and watch television and movies. Bit by bit, they come to understand themselves as males and females, which influences how they play and dress and talk and relate to other people.

And all is well in the neighborhood—until puberty hits like a flash flood and kids are up to their hips in hormones and high water.

Chubby boys grow angular; their voices crack and drop, muscles mass and occa-sionally cramp in places where there didn't even used to be *places*, hair sprouts like patches of grass, unanticipated erections ambush them by day and erotic dreams pro-duce involuntary ejaculations of semen by night. It is, by any standard, a crazy time to be a boy.

Skinny girls find their straight lines replaced by curving hips and bellies; their breasts bud and grow—evenly, they hope; they experience unexpected attention from males much older than themselves; hair grows on them too—though generally not as densely as on their brothers; and girls cross their fingers, hoping against hope that they'll be safe at home when they menstruate the first time. These are exceedingly strange days for girls morphing into women.

Such explosive change blows sexual perceptions all over the map. Some kids seem utterly unself-conscious about their sexuality. Others are conspicuously self-aware.

In the locker room, one boy saunters to the shower wearing nothing but a smile and a towel around his neck. The boy at the next locker wraps his towel around his waist like a kilt and holds it carefully lest he fall prey to a towel snatcher roaming the aisles of metal lockers. On the way, he passes a kid who doesn't need a towel because there's no way he's going near the shower.

In the classroom, a girl, dressed for comfort, is oblivious to the boy who sits behind her, transfixed by the curve of her shoulder. The girl in front of that girl is dressed to get attention and seems fully aware of her effect on boys—"She ain't got much," another girl whispers to her friend, "but it's all out there where they can get a look at it." At the back of the room, for reasons that are private and painful, another girl wears baggy clothes to hide her sexuality.

And so it goes in adolescence; the unconscious and the hyperconscious, question-ing, defining, and redefining their sexual identity.

What do kids want to know about their sexual identity?

> *Sexual identity* is how you experi-ence your sexuality—what you think of it and how you feel about it. This has a lot to do with hor-mones, but it's also shaped by how you're treated by family, friends, and culture.

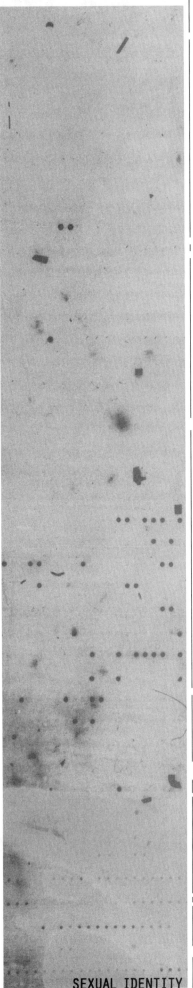

Well...ask around to be sure, but here's a short list of things kids everywhere seem to wonder:

- Am I normal?
- Am I gay?
- Are my sexual responses normal?
- Why do I get nervous around people of the other gender?
- Why do I get turned on so easily?
- Could I turn gay?
- Do I get turned on like other people?
- Why do I feel guilty about my sexuality?
- Am I a sex fiend?

This list hasn't changed much in the last 50 years. (Curiosity about homosexuality may have escalated a bit—kids generally talk about homosexuality more comfortably than their parents did back in their day. Other than that, the list looks about the same.)

The church's response to these questions hasn't changed much either. Christians who sit down for reasonable, biblically informed conversations about sexuality are few and far between. Half the church gets laryngitis when kids ask about these things. The other half talks louder.

Some people are just plain uncomfortable talking about sexuality. So they answer a question with a question:

"Whadaya mean, 'do you get turned on like other people?' You're not supposed to get turned on at all!"

"Why in the world would you even ask if you could turn into...one of those?"

One of our dirty little secrets is that Christians don't always agree on the subject of sexuality. In fact, Christians can be downright disagreeable on the subject.

Take gender roles, for instance.

Some Christians believe being male means one thing and one thing only. And being female means the exact opposite. So, for them, there are male jobs (thinking, heavy lifting, bringing home the bacon) and female jobs (cooking the bacon, cleaning, bearing and raising children) because that's the way God likes it. Anybody who crosses the behavioral divide has some explaining to do.

Other Christians believe the only differences between men and women are cultural, and therefore nonbiblical, if not frankly *un*biblical. They believe we invent what it means to act like women and men, culture by culture, as we go along. As far as those folks are concerned, gender is defined by plumbing and wiring, but behavior isn't—men can nurture without being feminine, and women can think without being masculine.

People in these two camps have been known to wonder if people in the other camp are even Christians.

Or take homosexuality.

- Some Christians believe homosexuality is a perversion, plain and simple—like sacrificing babies to Molech.
- Some believe homosexuality is a complex sin—like alcohol dependency.
- Some believe homosexuality is a biological abnormality—a mutant gene.
- Some believe homosexuality is a normal genetic trait—like blond hair.
- Some believe homosexuality is a lifestyle choice—like voting Republican.

Jam all those opinions in one room and things get pretty noisy. Or very quiet. For a lot of Christians, it's easier to not have the conversation at all.

That's a mistake. Maybe this goes without saying, but if we don't address kids' questions about sexual identity, someone else will. In fact, someone else is; loud and late into the night.

So we'd better.

reflect a moment...

Think about your sexual identity when you were eight years old.

Q: What did you believe it meant to be a woman?

Q: What did you believe it meant to be a man?

Fast-forward to age 15.

Q: How did your ideas about manhood change from childhood? What do you think influenced those changes?

Q: How did your ideas about womanhood change from childhood? What do you think influenced those changes?

Fast-forward to the present.

Q: List the most important things you believe contribute to authentic masculinity. How did you reach these conclusions?

Q: List the most important things you believe contribute to authentic femininity. How did you reach those conclusions?

Q: Are there things you believed as a child about your sexual identity that you no longer believe today? Spend some time thinking, writing, or talking with someone about that.

Q: Do you have unanswered questions about sexual identity? Spend some time thinking, writing, or talking with someone about that.

Q: If you had just one hour to talk with kids about sexual identity, what would you try to communicate?
  • Why do you think that's so important?
  • How would you try to communicate during that hour?

In our own words

SEX ID

VIDEO

How our sexual identity is formed. Introduce and show the video clip.

Q: What stands out the most for you in this video? Why do you think that's important?

Q: Do you identify with the people in the video? Talk about that.

Q: With what did you most strongly agree or disagree in the video? Why?

Q: Do you think the girl is finished with her sexual experimentation? Why?
- If you were a close friend, what would you have said to her when she said she was getting married? Why?
- What challenges do you think she'll face in the future? Why?

Q: Do these stories shed any light on how sexual identity is formed? Talk about that.

Although all sorts of forces are involved in forming our sexual identity, it seems that four of the major shaping forces are our genetic makeup, our experiences past and present, our families, and God. We're going to look at all four of these forces to try to figure out how they've molded us, and what we can do about it.

□ case studies

NATURE, NURTURE, OR BOTH

Is it because of my parents' DNA or the way they raised me?

For years, scientists have been debating the question of nature or nurture in human identity in general and sexual identity specifically. The debate seems to swirl around this key question: Am I the way I am because of the genes that I inherited from my parents, or because of the environment I grew up in, or some combination of the two? I'm going to read two true stories; hopefully, they'll illustrate some of the complex issues involved in this debate.

There was once an infant boy who, while being circumcised, was involved in a tragic accident that destroyed his penis. According to common medical practice, "in instances of extensive penile damage to infants it is standard to recommend rearing the male as a female."

This meant that this little boy's doctors built him a vagina because it's easier to do this than to rebuild a penis. His parents raised him as a female and never told him that he was actually born male. However, when he reached his teenage years, he knew something was wrong and subsequently switched to living as a male. According to the latest reports he is married to a woman, is raising three stepchildren, and is quite happy being male.

Q: Do you think the doctors were justified in making these changes after the accident?

Q: Be serious now. If you males among us were involved in an accident like the one above, would you rather live as a male with no penis or as a female with a fake vagina? Why?

"It can never be satisfied, the mind, never. Wallace Stevens wrote that, and in the long run he was right. The mind wants to live forever, or to learn a very good reason why not. The mind wants the world to return its love, or its awareness; the mind wants to know all the world and all eternity, and God. The mind's sidekick, however, will settle for two eggs over easy.

The dear stupid body is as easily satisfied as a spaniel. And, incredibly, the simple spaniel can lure the brawling mind to its dish. It is everlastingly funny that the proud, metaphysically ambitious, clamoring mind will hush if you give it an egg.

—Annie Dillard
in Teaching a Stone to Talk: Expeditions and Encounters (HarperCollins)

"Sex Reassignment at Birth: A Long Term Review and Clinical Implications," Milton Diamond, Ph.D., and H. Keith Sigmundson, M.D., *Archives of Pediatrics and Adolescent Medicine*, March 1997.

Q: Why do you think this sex reassignment did not work?
- What does this suggest about the way our biology, specifically whether we're genetically male or female, influences us?

Q: This is an example of someone whose environment tried to change him but failed. Can you think of any other instances where a person's environment tried to change him but failed?

Aaron was an 11-year-old boy who had normal feelings for pretty girls his age. He grew up in a middle-class house with two parents who loved each other a lot. From as far back as he could remember he had been going to church with his family and, even at this young age, knew he was a strong believer in Jesus. That is, until one day he accidentally walked into his mother's bedroom closet while she was naked.

As a reflex action, Aaron's mother slammed the closet door shut, and in the process jammed Aaron's fingers in the door. This was the first time he had seen a female naked, and the association between his mother's panic and his crushed fingers scarred him for life. He says that from that moment on he could never look at a female body without feeling pain. Aaron now lives as a homosexual who struggles with his relationship with Jesus.

Q: Do you think Aaron was genetically born or environmentally made a homosexual?

Q: Do you think it's possible that Aaron would have ended up as a gay man without this incident? Why or why not?

Q: Aaron's sexual identity was drastically altered by something that happened in the course of his life. Do you know anyone whose sexual identity has been shaped by incidents in their life?

Q: Aaron's story focuses on environmental influences. Other stories we hear are from people who say they never remember a time when they weren't more attracted to people of the same gender. They believe that's because they are somehow biologically gay. What do you think of that?
- Some Christians respond to the argument that homosexuality couldn't be biologically determined because God would not make someone that way. What do you think of this response?

Let's compare these two stories. The first was the story of someone who was born a certain way and his environment tried to change him, but it seems that his genetics won out. The second was a story of a man who was a born a certain way and an emotional trauma in his environment did change him.

discussion starter
LIKE FATHER, LIKE SON

Perhaps more than any other factor, our families shape our sexual identity.

Q: Kids learn from their families the things that establish, reinforce, or challenge their sexual identity (for example, boys are tough). What are some things the following relationships teach us about our sexual identity? (You don't have to go through all of them, you can select what you consider the most applicable.)

- father to son
- father to daughter
- mother to daughter
- mother to son

As we just admitted, there are a host of forces involved in forming sexual identity. However, we've chosen to focus on only four: biology, environment, family, and God. We wish we could narrow it down further, but given the wide assortment of social science and natural science research, we felt it would be intellectually dishonest to reduce it even further. If you would rather focus on just a few of these forces, by all means, please do. But we do hope that you'll join with us in presenting God as the ultimate potter who shapes us, the clay.

This discussion just scratches the surface of the issue of homosexuality. If you want—or if your students want—more on the topic, see **The "H" Word** (page 45).

As many as 125,000 teenagers each year say they are homeless—kicked out of their homes—because they are gay. About one-third of adolescent suicide attempts are by gay and lesbian teenagers. Ten percent of gay teens report being physically abused by family members.
—"20/20," ABC newsmagazine (September 13, 1999)

If your students are using *What (Almost) Nobody Will Tell You about Sex,* you can direct them to **Like Father, Like Son** (page 23).

YOU'LL NEED

- copies of **Like Father, Like Son** (page 50), one per student
- pencils

- brother to brother or sister to sister
- brother to sister or sister to brother
- cousins
- aunts and uncles
- step-parents

Q: What are the most helpful messages about sexual identity you've gotten from your family?

Q: What are the least helpful messages about sexual identity you've gotten from your family?

Q: What are some things you've learned about sexual identity from your family that you intend to pass on to your children?

Q: What have you learned about sexual identity from your family that you would rather not pass on to your children? Talk about that.

For even more provocative reflection or discussion, use the questions from **Like Father, Like Son** (page 57 in this book) in a large group, small group, or individual setting.

It's true that our genes, our environment, and our families impact our understanding of sexuality. But could it also be true that God wants to have the most say in the way we develop as sexual beings?

word from God

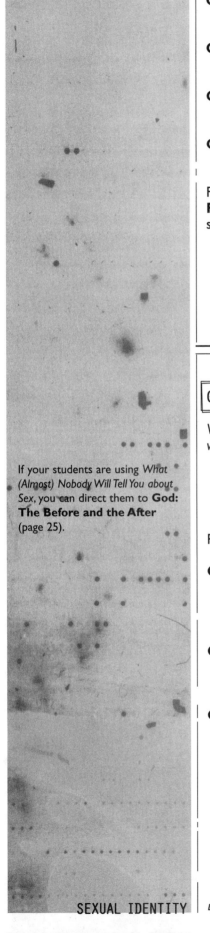

If your students are using *What (Almost) Nobody Will Tell You about Sex*, you can direct them to **God: The Before and the After** (page 25).

— Bible study —
GOD: THE BEFORE AND THE AFTER

Who we were before a relationship with God and who we are after we have a relationship with him can—or maybe even should—be pretty different.

In order to figure out God's influence on our sexual identity, we also must check out the effect a relationship with him has in our lives overall.

Read Romans 1:18-32 aloud.

Q: Given the people you know who don't have a relationship with God yet, how do you feel about Paul's label of them as wicked, evil, greedy, and depraved?
- Do you think it fits them or not?
- Would they agree with you or not? Talk about that.

Q: What do you believe about Paul's connection between following the sinful desires of the heart in verse 24 and the resulting shameful lusts that he describes in verses 26-28?

Q: In verse 21, Paul mentions that "they knew God," and yet here he goes on and on talking about all of their sin. Many biblical scholars believe Paul means they knew God in the sense of seeing his hand in creation (verse 20) but did not have a personal relationship with him. Do you think it's possible to get a glimpse of God from his creation?
- If so, why would someone continue to rebel against God?

Paul isn't mincing words here. He's saying that before we know Jesus, we're really messed up. Thank God (literally) that's not the end of the story.

Read 2 Corinthians 5:17 aloud.

Q: What a great verse! When we enter into a relationship with Jesus, the bad stuff we just read about in Romans is wiped away. Gone just like that. In what ways would that make a difference in a person's sexual identity?

Q: Okay, but wait a minute. If we're "new creations," why is it that many of us still struggle with sin issues—sexual stuff in particular?

Q: How is it possible that the reality that we are brand-new creations in Christ coexists with the ever-present reality that we are sinful, broken, struggling believers?

Q: Paul seems to address this very tension in Romans 7:14-28. He seems fully aware of the inner struggle between doing what's right and what's wrong—and yet points to a rescuer in Romans 7:24. Who is that rescuer?

Q: It's true that Jesus rescues us from our sin when we ask him to take over our lives and be our Savior and Lord. But how do we need him to rescue us from our sin and sexual struggles even after we have committed our lives to him?

the last word

─ discussion and writing activity
| A NEW CREATION |

Being a new creation has already transformed us, and yet we still need God to continue to transform us.

Begin this activity with these comments.

> **Justin McRoberts wrote a song on his album *Reason for Living* called "Galatians 2:20." Listen to some of the words:**
>
> > **I have sinned, I have broken your heart
> > I have strayed from the path that you laid down for me Lord,
> > and what can I do
> > I am the problem and I am helpless in myself**
>
> **Sounds pretty bleak, doesn't it—a little bit like Romans chapter 1, if you ask me. But the song goes on,**
>
> > **I have been crucified with Christ and no longer live
> > I am a new creation now**
>
> **This is the beauty of the message that Jesus came to bring: once we were so bad, but now, because of what he did, we are brand-spanking new—even if we don't always feel or understand it. Our sexual identity has to flow from the understanding that we are new creations in Jesus.**

Q: The first three forces we looked at in forming our sexual identity are our biology, our environment, and our families. How would you rank these in order of most influential to least influential?

Q: What about God, the fourth force? Where does he fit in your ranking?

Q: Some would argue that if we're struggling with our sexual identity, God can bring us healing and wholeness, no matter what our problems or struggles are. Do you agree?

If any man is in Christ, he is a new creation (some assembly required).

Justin McRoberts, *Reason for Living,* (5 Minute Walk Records)

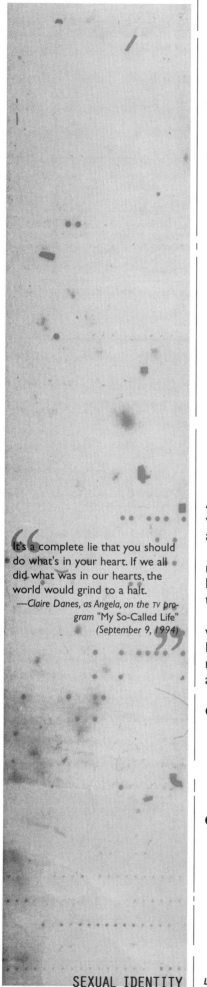

I'm going to read a handful of issues that are part of our sexual identity. As I read each one, I'm going to ask three questions:

Q: Would you recommend that this person try to change this issue, or is it okay as it's described?

Q: If you'd recommend some sort of change, how do you think God might want to be involved in that?

Q: If you'd recommend some sort of change, and this person was a friend of yours, how do you think you might want to be involved in that?

- **A girl who is a tomboy and yet feels like maybe she should act a little more feminine at times**
- **A guy who feels a bit like a sissy and would like to be a bit more like one of the guys**
- **A girl who's afraid of being abandoned by guys so she doesn't date at all**
- **Someone who's ashamed of her body**
- **Someone who uses his body as a tool to get what he wants**
- **A girl who can't stop thinking about the guy who sits next to her in math**
- **A guy who can't stop thinking about the guy who sits next to him in that same math class**

Let's get even more personal. How about you? What issues are you dealing with? If you'd like to change how you're handling these issues, how would you like God to help you change?

As you ask the questions described below, invite students to write down how they were before they accepted Jesus' rescue from their sin, the difference in their life after that point, and finally, the struggles or questions they still are working through.

If most of your students are not already Christians, or if you're not sure, this might be a great chance to invite them to consider who they are without him, who he is, and what it would take for them to have eternal life with him—plus a way better life in the present.

If you have a pretty even mix between Christians and non-Christians, you might want to challenge them to face off in a rousing match of tug-of-war. Just kidding. Instead, it might be more appropriate to ask the following questions in an environment conducive to personal reflection, with plenty of time for students to really think and be still before God.

Q: If you have already asked Jesus to rescue you from your sins and be your Savior and Lord, how has that made a difference in your sexual identity?
- What sexual struggles and questions do you still need Jesus' help with?
- It's been said that sin is often a result of pride or laziness. How might either of these be keeping you from fully experiencing what it means to be a new creation with a healthy sexual identity?

Q: If you haven't asked Jesus to rescue you from your sins and be your Savior and Lord, what questions or unresolved issues do you have that keep you from doing so?
- How do you think allowing him to rescue you would impact your view of yourself and your sexual identity?

In other ~~words~~

┌─ video discussion starter ──────────────────────────┐
│ BOYS WILL BE ____ AND GIRLS WILL BE ____ │──────── VIDEO
└──┘

What do girls think of guys? What do guys think of girls? Wouldn't you like to know?
After playing the **"Boys Will Be _____ and Girls Will Be _____"** video clip,
ask questions like the following.

Q: How confusing do you find the opposite gender?
- ☐ Not confusing at all
- ☐ Pretty perplexing
- ☐ Absolutely mind-blowing

Q: How different do you think the two genders are?
- ☐ No different
- ☐ A bit different
- ☐ Fairly different
- ☐ Way different

Q: Several differences were mentioned in the video. Let's see whether or not you
agree with what was highlighted.
- • Is it really true that girls are more emotional?
- • How about that girls are more serious about their relationships?
- • Do you think guys are really less mature?

Q: One guy on the video mentions a double standard for girls and guys. Do you
agree that this double standard exists? If so, what are some examples?

Q: Is it true that guys evaluate girls primarily by their physical appearance while girls
focus more on guys' internal qualities?

Q: Girls, what other words or phrases would you use to describe guys not
mentioned on the video?
- • Guys, what other words or phrases would you use to describe girls not
mentioned on the video?

Q: Girls, how do the words from the video—as well as what the guys just shared—
affect your sexual identity?
- • Guys, how do the words from the video—as well as what the girls just
shared—affect your sexual identity?

┌─ discussion starter ─────────────┐
│ THAT'S GOTTA HURT │────────────────────────────────────
└──────────────────┘

Tragic circumstances can affect our sexual identity.

Q: It's amazing how powerful spoken words are. When Tiger Woods was growing
up, his father instilled in him the vision that one day he would be not just the
greatest African-American golfer, but the greatest golfer ever. He is well on his
way to becoming that very person. On the other hand, there are many people
who grow up with negative verbal abuse that scars them forever. Without naming
names, do you know anyone who has suffered from negative verbal abuse? Can
you tell that person's story?

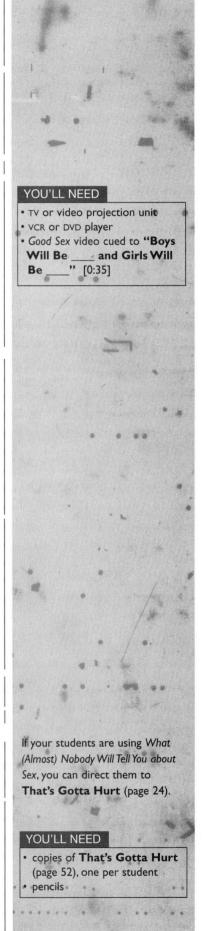

YOU'LL NEED
- TV or video projection unit
- VCR or DVD player
- *Good Sex* video cued to **"Boys Will Be ____ and Girls Will Be ____"** [0:35]

If your students are using *What (Almost) Nobody Will Tell You about Sex*, you can direct them to **That's Gotta Hurt** (page 24).

YOU'LL NEED
- copies of **That's Gotta Hurt** (page 52), one per student
- pencils

Q: With this in mind, what effect do you think verbal and emotional abuse might have on a person's sexual identity? Talk about that.

Q: What effect do you think physical disability might have on a person's sexual identity? Talk about that.

Q: What effect do you think sexual molestation might have on a person's sexual identity?

Q: What effect do you think rape might have on a person's sexual identity? Talk about that.

Q: What effect do you think incest might have on a person's sexual identity?

Q: Can you think of any other circumstances that might have a real effect on our sexual identity?

Q: Do you have any close friends or family who have suffered in any of these ways? How do you think they cope, if at all, with the effects?

To help students further understand the way their sexual identity has been affected by painful experiences, use the questions included in **That's Gotta Hurt** (page 52 in this book) for large or small group discussions, as well as for individual, personal reflection.

— list-making game —
TALKING DIRTY

How we talk about sex impacts how we view it (caution—this discussion is best for mature groups).

Ask your students to think about or write the terms people in their culture use to talk about sex, and if you'd like, write them on the whiteboard or index cards. Then ask them the following questions.

Q: Are the majority of these words common or uncommon in the places where you hang out?

Q: Which of these terms are offensive to you? Why?

Q: Do you think the language a person uses affects his or her sexual identity? Why or why not?

To help your students more fully consider the impact of words and actions on their sexual identity, use the questions from Talking Dirty (page 53 in this book) for large group discussion, smaller group processing, or individual reflection.

YOU'LL NEED

• list-making materials. Some combination of the following: a whiteboard, markers, different colored index cards, or sheets of butcher paper hung on the wall. You get the idea. (Or, if you wish, just let this one be a mental exercise.)
• copies of **Talking Dirty** (page 53), one per student
• pencils

Don't do this exercise if you can't do it in good conscience. And please don't get mad at us for including it. It's just, when you ask your group to think of or write down the words used to describe sex in their culture, they're going to think of some words we all wish weren't as common as they are these days. If we take language seriously—and we do—those words affect the way people understand and feel about sex—even if that understanding and those feelings are unexamined. We think it's a good idea to examine them. But if your conscience—or your boss—won't allow you to go there, please let yourself and us off the hook and just skip this page.

THE "H" WORD

What we believe and feel about homosexuality. (Buckle up!)

Q: Which statement best describes your opinion?

- I believe homosexuals are born, not made—it runs in the family genes.
- I believe homosexuals are made by their environments, not born.
- I believe homosexuals are homosexual for many reasons, not just one.
- I believe homosexuals have perverted thinking.
- I believe homosexuality is a birth defect, like spina bifida or cystic fibrosis.
- I don't think I know why some people are homosexual.
- The reason I believe some people are homosexuals is _____.

Choose three students that replied to each of these responses who are willing to complete one of these statements:

- I agreed that homosexuals are born, not made, because...
- I agreed that homosexuals are made, not born, because...
- I agreed that I don't know why some people are homosexual because...

Q: How many of you actually know someone who describes himself or herself as homosexual?

Q: For those of you who responded in the affirmative, how does that person feel about his or her sexuality?

Q: Are you well acquainted with someone who doesn't describe himself or herself as homosexual but you think probably is?
- If so, what makes you think that person is a homosexual?

Q: Homosexual relationships seem to be getting an increasing amount of attention in today's culture. Do you think that sometimes in our society—and maybe even among some of your friends—it has become kinda cool to be gay?
- If you agree, why do you think it is this way?

Q: What do you believe about homosexual relationships being more acceptable today than they used to be?
- How do you think Scripture speaks to this issue? Do you know any passages offhand that relate to homosexuality?

If your students need some hints on biblical passages, try pointing them to Genesis 19:1-17, Leviticus 18:1-30, Romans 1:18-2:15, and 1 Corinthians 6:9-11.

Q: How do those Scripture verses affect your view of homosexuality?

Q: It's been said that, given the other sins described in many of these passages, homosexuality is no worse than any other sin, including heterosexual lust. What do you think of that argument?

Q: Do you think there's a difference between homosexual curiosity and homosexual identity? Talk about that.
- How about between homosexual tendencies and acting on those tendencies?

> So what started as an entertainment magazine quickly became a handbook for men, and the message was that you could live a moral and ethical life that is not simply defined as being a husband and a father.
>
> —Hugh Hefner, Playboy founder, describing the early days of his magazine (Details, April 1993)

If your students are using *What (Almost) Nobody Will Tell You about Sex*, you can direct them to **The "H" Word** (page 34).

YOU'LL NEED

- copies of **The "H" Word** (page 54) or **The Grass Is Browner** (page 54/55), one per student
- pencils

We bring up the question of homosexuality because we know your students wonder about it. We do not claim to have all the answers, but we hope this discussion will be helpful to you, and more importantly, to your students. Since not all denominations agree on this issue, nor do all churches within a denomination, nor do all people within a single church, it seems likely that your group of students will be somewhat fractured in their opinions also.

At the time of this writing, the research regarding the influence of biological forces in the development of sexual identity (especially homosexual identity) is conflicting.

Read Ezekiel 16:46-52 with your students, then use the following questions for discussion. You may want to familiarize yourself with Sodom's escapades in Genesis 18-19 (either ahead of time and summarize the events for your students, or together as a group during the discussion).

Q: What do you think is the big idea here? Talk about that.

A thought about Ezekiel 16:46-52—

> **God said the people of Israel (that's his subject in this passage) were so bad they made the wrongdoers in Samaria and Sodom look like Girl Scouts. Most of Ezekiel 16 is an extended metaphor in which God rescues and nurtures Israel as an infant child, raises her to adulthood, and then marries her as an act of committed love—only to watch her turn into a raging sex addict who sleeps with everyone but her own husband. Despite her great beauty, she actually pays men to sleep with her, driving her husband mad. It's a vivid picture.**
>
> **Here's the kicker. With this image of sexual debauchery and craziness, God says his beloved Israel is acting worse than Sodom ever did—but oddly enough, God doesn't say a word about sex when he talks about Sodom in Ezekiel 16. God's beef with Sodom is that she was arrogant, overfed, and unconcerned. She failed to help the poor. She was haughty and disgusting. But God doesn't mention sodomy. This is not to say the violent lustiness of the men of Sodom in Genesis 18 and 19 wasn't a big deal. The results speak for themselves. But sex is not what Ezekiel uses to make his point about how bad they were.**

Q: What do you think about these thoughts on Ezekiel 16? Talk about that.
  • Where do you agree? Talk about that.
  • Where do you disagree? Talk about that.

Q: Why do you think Sodom is more widely known for Genesis 18 and 19 than Ezekiel 16? Talk about that.

Q: As one preacher puts it, for every person who struggles with the sins of Sodom, there are nine who struggle with the sins of Jerusalem. What do you think that means?

Q: Some churches have the reputation for being unwelcoming to homosexuals, insisting that they change their lifestyles before they become a part of the community. Other churches welcome homosexuals just as they are and don't require that they change their behavior or lifestyle at all. Still others welcome homosexuals into the church community but exclude them from leadership. What do you think of these three positions? What do you believe God thinks of them?
  • If you were in charge of a church, what would you hope would be its approach to homosexuals?

Q: Some Christians believe that ministry to homosexuals begins with loving them and getting to know them. Others believe it begins with telling them that they're disobeying God. What do you think of these two starting points?
  • If you had a friend who was homosexual—and many of you do—how would you want to start ministering to that friend?

To dive even further and more personally into the topic of homosexuality and judgmentalism, use the questions found on **The "H" Word** (page 54 in this book) or **The Grass Is Browner** (page 55 in this book) as material for large or small group discussion, or individual personal reflection.

It's taken a long time to realize that God is not the enemy of my enemies—he's not the enemy of his enemies.
—attributed to Martin Niemuller, German pastor imprisoned by Nazis

FRUIT: A MANLY MEAL OR A FEMININE DELIGHT?

How the fruit of the Spirit shows up in our lives after we have a personal relationship with God, regardless of our gender.

Read Galatians 5:22-23 with your students, then use the following questions for discussion.

Q: In this passage Paul lists the well-known fruit of the Spirit. Do you think of the attributes in Galatians 5:22-23 as more masculine or more feminine?

FRUIT	MORE FEMININE BECAUSE...	MORE MASCULINE BECAUSE...	BOTH FEMININE AND MASCULINE BECAUSE...
Love			
Joy			
Peace			
Patience			
Kindness			
Goodness			
Faithfulness			
Gentleness			
Self-Control			

Q: Do you think most people in our culture seem confused, or rather clear about what's masculine and what's feminine?

Read Galatians 3:26-28 with your students.

Jesus combined what we call masculine and feminine traits in a comfortable balance of humanness. He hugged children and spoke up for them in Mark 10:13-16; he got physical with merchants who exploited poor people in the temple in John 2:13-22; he was tough on people who were full of themselves in John 5:41-47; he cried over the grief of a friend in John 11:35. Jesus was not a stereotypical, testosterone-crazed man and he wasn't a sissy. In a culture where children were disposable and women would have been second-class citizens if they'd been allowed to be citizens at all, Jesus respected children and treated women as equals. And the spirit of Jesus, the Holy Spirit, produces fruit in every believer's life as if gender had nothing to do with anything.

The fruit of the Spirit is love, joy, peace, patience, kindness, goodness, faithfulness, gentleness, and self-control. God's Spirit nullifies "boys will be boys" and "women—can't live with 'em, can't live without 'em." The Holy Spirit replaces roughness with gentleness and transforms compulsiveness into self-control. Not quickly, perhaps, but inevitably.

This is not to say there's no difference between men and women, only that the differences have nothing to do with character, nothing to do with giftedness or fruitfulness, nothing to do with anything that matters in the next life. Does this make sense in our culture

YOU'LL NEED

- copies of **Fruit: A Manly Meal or a Feminine Delight?** (page 56), one per student
- pencils

If your students are using *What (Almost) Nobody Will Tell You about Sex,* you can direct them to **Fruit: A Manly Meal or a Feminine Delight?** (page 30).

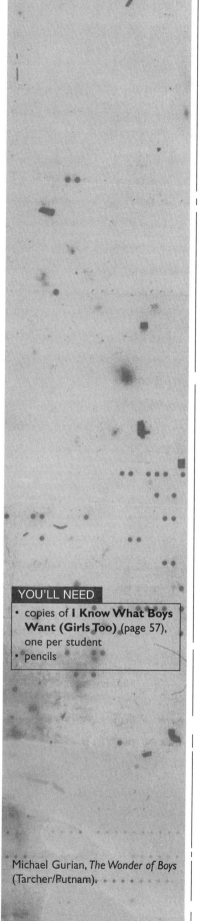

where people are stereotyped from the moment of birth? Not really. But so what? As Jesus put it to Nicodemus in John 3:8, "The wind blows wherever it pleases. You hear its sound, but you cannot tell where it comes from or where it is going. So it is with everyone born of the Spirit." The people of God—male and female—are freaks in the world's eyes. We don't fit cultural norms because we're coming from another place. Our passports are issued in the kingdom of heaven where we are—every one of us by God's grace—naturalized citizens.

All of which is to say that in our culture, women may be considered masculine and men may be thought feminine for exhibiting characteristics that are merely godly. And it breaks my heart—on those days when it doesn't make me angry—that these characterizations are about as common inside the family of God as outside. We can't control what outsiders say about us, but shame on us for choosing cultural stereotypes over biblical models of transformation and growth. That's just plain wrong.

Q: In what ways does our society force gender norms on us?

Q: In Galatians 3:26-28, is Paul saying that when we become followers of Jesus Christ, we lose those things that make us male and female?

Q: What do you think he's getting at?

Q: What do you think we have to gain or lose by treating each other *first* as humans made in God's image, and *then* as male and female? Talk about that.

Q: What do you think we have to gain or lose by accepting and passing on the gender norms of our culture? Talk about that.

To help students further examine their own perspectives on femininity, masculinity, fruit of the Spirit, and the relationship between them all, use the questions found on **Fruit: A Manly Meal or a Feminine Delight?** (page 56 in this book) in a large group, a small group, or as a tool for individual reflection.

---

discussion starter

I KNOW WHAT BOYS WANT (GIRLS TOO)

Some of the top questions boys and girls are asking about their sexual identity.

Michael Gurian is a therapist with a lot of young clients. Here's his list of things boys want to know.

- How do I control myself?
- Why do I get so nervous around girls? Does everyone—even athletic stars?
- How come he's got more hair than I do?
- Why do girls manipulate me so well?
- Will I ever get pubic hair?
- Am I big enough?
- How can I get more sex?
- Am I gay?
- Why do I feel ashamed of myself so much?

Q: Do you think there's any question missing from this list?

Q: Most boys don't ask a therapist to answer these questions. Where do you think most boys get their answers?

Michael Gurian, *The Wonder of Boys* (Tarcher/Putnam).

YOU'LL NEED

- copies of **I Know What Boys Want (Girls Too)** (page 57), one per student
- pencils

Q: What questions do you think girls would love to ask about themselves?

Q: Where do you think most girls get their answers?

Q: What do you think is the one thing that boys most want to know about girls?

Q: What do you think is the one thing that girls most want to know about boys?

Conclude this discussion by distributing copies of **I Know What Boys Want (Girls Too)** (page 57 in this book) and pencils to students. After giving them five to 10 minutes to individually write down their answers, invite them to huddle into small groups with two other students and share answers to two of the six questions (they pick which two).

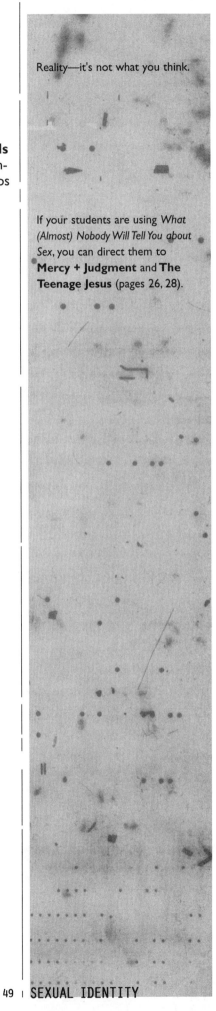

Reality—it's not what you think.

If your students are using *What (Almost) Nobody Will Tell You about Sex*, you can direct them to **Mercy + Judgment** and **The Teenage Jesus** (pages 26, 28).

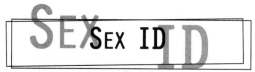

Reflect on these questions.

Q: What messages have you gotten about your sexual identity from the following?

- family

- classmates

- teachers

- church or youth group or Christian events

- coaches

- employers

- television or movies

- books

- magazines

- music

- Internet

- radio

Q: Have any of those messages helped you?

Q: Have any of those messages damaged you?

Q: What voices consistently affirm your sexual identity?

Q: What voices consistently challenge your sexual identity?

Q: What are some things that you can do to gain God's perspective on some of these other voices that you are listening to?

LIKE FATHER, LIKE SON

Reflect on these questions.

Q: Do you think the sexual identity messages you're getting from your family are different from what other families give?

Q: What are the most helpful messages about sexual identity you've gotten from your family?
   • What are the least helpful messages about sexual identity you've gotten from your family?

Q: What have you learned about sexual identity from your family that you intend to pass on to your children?
   • What have you learned about sexual identity from your family that you would rather not pass on to your children? Talk about that.

Q: Is there anything about your sexual identity you wish you could talk about with someone? If so, what is that thing that you would like to discuss—and what do you think you have to gain or lose by having that conversation?

THAT'S GOTTA HURT

Reflect on the following questions.

Q: To what degree would you say your sexual identity has been influenced by the following?

	zero degree	to some degree	a great degree
physical disability			
verbal and emotional abuse			
violent physical abuse			
sexual molestation			
rape			
incest			
you name it: _____			

Q: If you've been the victim of any of these wrongs, who knows about it besides you and the person or persons responsible?

☐ Nobody else knows.
- If this is true, do you think it might be better to let someone in on this? What do you have to gain or lose?

☐ I have great support from people who can really do something to help.
- If this is true, how did they find out about your need?
- Talk about what those people do that is helpful.
- What have you learned from them about helping people in pain?

☐ Other people know, but they couldn't—or wouldn't—do anything to help.
- If this is true, how did they find out about your need?
- Why do you think they couldn't or wouldn't help?
- Describe how you feel about not getting the help you need.

Q: Do you think you know someone whose sexual identity has been influenced by any of the factors we're talking about here? Check all that apply.

☐ physical disability   ☐ verbal and emotional abuse   ☐ physical abuse
☐ sexual molestation   ☐ rape   ☐ incest
☐ you name it: _____

Q: Do you believe you can do anything to help this person?

Q: As you finish this reflection, is there anything you think you need to do in response to what you've been thinking about?
- If so, what do you think you have to gain or lose by taking that next step?

TALKING DIRTY

Reflect on these questions.

Q: Would you say your view of sex is more positive or negative than the view of people you hang out with? Why?

Very negative	About the same	Very positive

Q: Do you feel like people you're with or the environment you're in tries to bring down or raise your view of sex?

Q: Who do you think has the most positive influence on your sexual identity? Why?
- What are some things you can do to get more of that positive influence in your life?
- How do your parents talk about sex? What impact do you believe that has on your view of sex?
- How do your friends talk about sex? What impact do you believe that has on your view of sex?

Reflect on these questions.

Q: Why do you think homosexuality is such a volatile issue in our culture?

Q: Do you believe there's any difference between homosexual curiosity and homosexual identity? If so, what is the difference?

Q: Have you had any homosexual curiosity?

Q: Have you had any homosexual experiences?

Q: If someone close to you said she thought she might be a homosexual, what would you say to her?

Q: If someone close to you said he no longer wanted to identify himself as a homosexual, what would you say to him?

Q: What questions do you have about homosexuality?

Q: To whom would you go to talk about those questions?

THE GRASS IS BROWNER

Q: It seems like when people get all huffy about other people's behavior, it's usually about things they don't have in common. For example, someone may get more upset about homosexuality (something he's never experienced) than pornography (something he understands quite well). Do you think this is a true observation?

Q: Have you ever been on the receiving end of this kind of thing—harshly judged by someone who experiences a different set of struggles than you do?

Q: Have you been on the judging end of that—being hard on someone whose issues you didn't understand while going easier on someone with whom you identified more closely?

Q: Do you wrestle with something that leaves you feeling isolated?
• If you have that kind of struggle, and if you were going to let someone in on it, do you think you know someone who might be a safe person?

Q: If you know someone struggling with an issue that isolates them, what do you think you could do to become a safe and helpful confidant for that individual?
• Take a moment to pray for that person right now.

FRUIT: A MANLY MEAL OR A FEMININE DELIGHT?

Reflect on these questions.

Q: Do you ever wonder if you're as masculine or as feminine as you're supposed to be?

Q: Who are the best models of masculinity you know?
• What makes their masculinity appealing?

Q: Who are the best models of femininity you know?
• What makes their femininity appealing?

Q: Do you generally think of anything on the list in Galatians 5:22-23 as seeming more masculine than feminine or vice versa? If so, which to you are the masculine and which are the more feminine? Why do you suppose those attributes seem more masculine or feminine to you?

Q: Think back on the past year. Which fruit of the Spirit would you say is more abundant in your life today than a year ago? How do you feel about that?

Q: Do you think any of the Spirit's fruit is less abundant in your life than a year ago? How do you feel about that?

Reflect on these questions.

Q: What questions did you have about your sexuality when you were younger?
- Where did you go for answers?
- How satisfied are you with the answers you got?

Q: What questions do you have about your sexuality now?
- Where do you go for answers?
- To whom can you go for help? What do you have to gain or lose by asking for help?

before you
teach this lesson...

Sex does not equal intimacy. Intimacy equals intimacy. What's so hard about that?

Well—maybe it's hard because most of us don't really know what intimacy means, let alone how to be intimate.

Intimacy grows between people who trust each other with their deepest natures. Intimacy rejects fakery and shortcuts. There's no such thing as instant intimacy. Instant attraction, yes. Instant crushes, of course. But real intimacy takes time. You can tell you're in an intimate relationship if you both choose being real instead of faking it, being warm instead of cool, being understanding instead of judging—not every day, maybe, but most of the time, for a long time.

The feelings that come with intimacy can be huge, spanning the distance from inexpressibly glad to unspeakably sad, from the hollow ache of separation to the giddy abandon of reunion.

But intimacy is not a feeling, it's a condition. Intimacy takes time and attention and energy. To some people, that sounds a lot like work. So sometimes people do things to *feel* intimate, even if they aren't really. It's rumored that some girls are interested in sex because it makes them feel intimate—and it's also rumored that some boys fake intimacy in order to get sex.

It doesn't take a genius to understand what happens when people pretend to be intimate. Intimacy Lite—less filling, but still intoxicating in sufficient quantities.

It also doesn't take a genius to understand why people might settle for Intimacy Lite. True intimacy is risky. Being intimate means facing the possibility of rejection and embarrassment. If I reveal the truth about me, I risk the possibility that you'll say, "Eww, that's creepy." Which, needless to say, is painful. And if you tell other people I'm creepy, the stakes rise to the level of humiliation, and who needs that?

That's why intimacy is so hard: because it's a high-risk investment. And everyone knows that Rule One of investing is *Don't risk more than you can afford to lose*.

So, after we get hurt a couple of times, most of us learn to lie back and play it safe, investing a little of our true selves but not enough to risk a serious loss.

It's a good strategy. Except for the fact that humans need intimacy—whether we want it or not.

Right from the start (Genesis 2:18), God declared that humans ought not to be alone; we need help to make it. God says, plain as day, it's not good for humans to be isolated. Most of us know instinctively that God is right about this. Dangerous as it is, what people crave, perhaps more than anything else, is authentic intimacy.

It turns out that sex is a handy substitute for authentic intimacy.

There's no question that sex feels intimate. Breathing the same air, sharing the same space, being *glued together* sexually is how the Bible puts it when it says two people are united as "one flesh" (Genesis 2:24; Matthew 19:5-6; Mark 10:7-8; 1 Corinthians 6:16; Ephesians 5:31—the words translated *cleave* in the King James and *united* in the NIV mean *to glue together*). It's hard to get any closer than that.

But when a relationship comes unglued, so do the feelings. Sometimes the people come apart as well. Here's how a tenth-grade friend expressed her loss:

**my heart is locked
the key is gone
one took the key first
but he mocked my inner strengths
and beauties**

Intimacy is being open, honest, vulnerable, trusting, caring, and giving with another person who treats you the same way.

Fool me once, shame on you; fool me twice, shame on me.

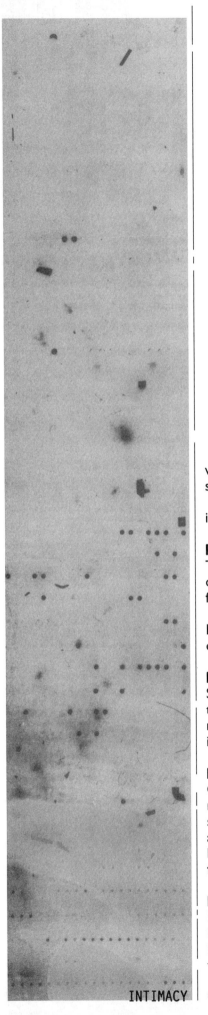

then he threw away my key
and left me open to all
many came
all went
finally I took the key
and locked me back up
not allowing anyone to enter,
and threw away the key
one kind person ventured
under the trash that had piled
high over my key
he was considerate enough
to find my key
which no one had time to find
he started to open me
but didn't get very far
then he left
like every one else in
this human world of
imperfection
I will not allow anyone
in my heart
for a long time

This is your heart.
This is your heart broken.
Any questions?

Do you ever wonder why dating—the way most of us do it—doesn't work very well? Why the shortest distance between a blissful crush and wishing you never met someone is going out with him or her?

Dating can be a messy business (this is just a general observation—skip this part if you think you're the exception to the rule). Here's how most dating breaks down.

PHASE ONE—GUESS WHO
The mess begins when someone—let's call her Sophie—tries to figure out what sort of person the sort of person she wants to go out with wants to go out with. Are you following this?

Generally, Sophie has someone in mind—Joaquin or Billy Joe or Shaquille or Haing, could be anyone—because he's cute or looks like he needs rescuing or whatever.

PHASE TWO—MASQUERADE
Sophie figures out what Haing wants and says, "I can be that." Then she fakes her way to romance. Sooner or later, directly or indirectly, Sophie tells a lie to maintain the masquerade. It's doomed from the start—anyone can see that. The only thing missing is the voice of that lady from the "Nick at Nite" laugh track saying, "Uh-oh!"

PHASE THREE—GETTING SERIOUS
Getting serious is easy to spot—just look for two high school juniors acting like married people, except they live with their parents. Neither can make plans without consulting the other. They cross the borders of married sexual behavior. They can't talk about where they'd like to be in five years without somebody getting their feelings hurt. They buy stuff together. Sophie finds it's easier to have sex (which makes her feel close, temporarily at least, to Haing) than talk seriously with him.

PHASE FOUR—THE CINDERELLA SYNDROME
Eventually, the clock strikes 12 and Sophie turns into the poor stepsister. It's humiliating and sad, and she feels she's lost something she can't replace. She's distracted (or intensely focused), she can't sleep (or can't wake up), she gains some weight (or loses weight rapidly). For a while, Sophie wonders if she'll make it. But, after a few weeks,

she thinks it's probably just as well because she never really enjoyed pretending to be a Cow-Punk-Choir-Girl-Skate-Rat anyway. Haing was a jerk—how could she not see that? Sophie makes a mental note not to get so emotionally involved next time. If there is a next time.

Then one day, out of the blue, Sophie wonders, again, what sort of person the sort of person she wants to go out with wants to go out with. You following this?

No wonder some people try to drain the emotion from sexuality.

But it doesn't work. This is the message of countless soap operas, sitcoms, movies and books, including the Bible. No matter what people say about casual sex, in the end, it's quite personal. If you don't believe it, keep watching.

Now here's a funny thing: for people who want to take the intimacy out of sex, we're awfully busy sexualizing intimacy these days. Many in our culture believe intimacy leads inevitably to sex. "You can't get that close to people without going farther," they say. And by *going farther*, they mean getting sexual. This is intimacy as foreplay, and it's highly toxic to otherwise healthy friendships. (Have you noticed how many people get sexually involved with their close friends...and how they tend to drift apart afterward?) There goes the possibility of friendship between men and women. Too bad.

The Bible describes us—Christians, at least—as brothers and sisters. Sorry, but there are things healthy brothers and sisters don't do, and it's not because they're not intimate. They've shared a bathroom, for goodness' sake. They've had the measles together. They've fought like cats and dogs, then made up because, underneath it all, they love each other. They've laid awake giggling on Christmas eve, too wired to sleep. They've nursed each other through tough times with Mom or Dad. That's fertile ground for intimacy, and it's the relational model for Christians in community. Sex screws that up something terrible.

Even same-gender intimacy is threatened by the assumption or fear that people can't get close without getting busy. Not everybody makes that assumption; not by a long shot. It's crazy and unfair. But it's there like a rumor, isolating people; making them uncomfortable and suspicious and separate. Again: too bad. It's not supposed to be like this. Because it's no good for people to be isolated. God said so.

> **John:** "You slept with her!?"
> **Richard:** "Don't worry; it wasn't intimate."
>
> —"*Ally McBeal*,"
> *Fox Television, May 15, 2000*

what's in this lesson...

reflect a moment...

To help your students most effectively, you need to make every effort to process your own sexual experiences, questions, and struggles. Here are some questions to get you thinking:

Q: When you were 15, what did you think intimacy meant?
• Where did you get those ideas?

Q: What do you believe intimacy means today?
  • How did you reach your conclusions?

Q: Describe your most intimate relationships, past and present.

Q: Have you experienced intimacy that seems unhealthy to you now?

Q: What has romance added or subtracted in your experience of intimacy?

Q: What are your future hopes for intimacy?

Q: If you had just one hour to talk with kids about intimacy, what would you try to communicate?
  • Why do you think that's so important?
  • If you were prevented from lecturing on the subject, how would you try to communicate during that hour?

If your students are using *What (Almost) Nobody Will Tell You about Sex,* you can direct them to **Intimacy** (page 39).

In our own words

— video opener
INTIMACY ────────────────────────────────── VIDEO

Some thoughts about intimacy—real and imagined.

After watching the video clip **"Intimacy"** with your students, lead the following discussion.

Q: What comment resonated with what you feel about intimacy?

Q: Where would you guess that some of these people got their ideas about intimacy?

Q: How would you define intimacy?

Q: How did you come up with that definition?
  • How is intimacy different than lust?

Q: Is intimacy really more of a *woman thing* than a *man thing*? Why or why not?

Q: Is there a difference between intimacy with the same gender and intimacy between genders? Explain what you think.

Q: Do you believe intimacy has to lead to sex?

ABSOLUTELY NOT BECAUSE...	MAYBE, MAYBE NOT BECAUSE...	ABSOLUTELY BECAUSE...

Q: Do you believe sex is the most intimate act that humans can perform?

ABSOLUTELY NOT BECAUSE...	MAYBE, MAYBE NOT BECAUSE...	ABSOLUTELY BECAUSE...

Q: What do you think you still have to learn about intimacy? Why?

To help students process the above questions, and a whole host of others, use the questions found on **Intimacy** (page 76 in this book) for large or small group reflection, or for personal reflection.

┌ live case study ┐
LOVE STORIES

Life-sized visual aids of long-term, intimate relationships.

Invite a couple whose marriage you admire to answer these questions. Brief them before they come in front of the group, asking that they be as real and honest as humanly possible. Ask them to please not preach, but to tell their stories directly and trust you to help student process the meaning.

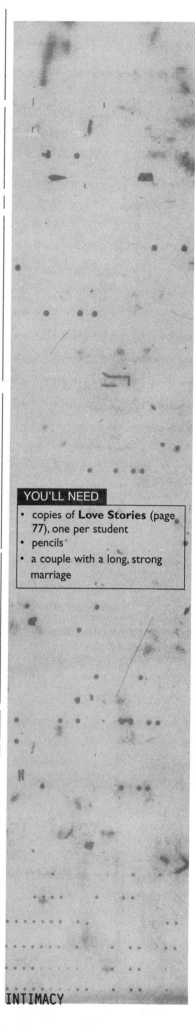

YOU'LL NEED
- copies of **Love Stories** (page 77), one per student
- pencils
- a couple with a long, strong marriage

Q: In under a minute, can you tell us how your love story began?

Q: What, if anything, did you share in common at the beginning of your relationship?

Q: How did you know at first that this was someone that you would like to see more of?

Q: How long into the relationship before you knew that this was the one?

Q: How did you find that out?

Q: What were the biggest struggles you had while you were dating? How did you overcome them?

Q: What did your love bring you that you didn't have before you met?

Q: Where were you when you proposed or got proposed to? On a scale of 1-10, 10 being the most, how romantic was it when this proposal took place?

Q: In what ways have you continued to grow intimate with each other since you were married?

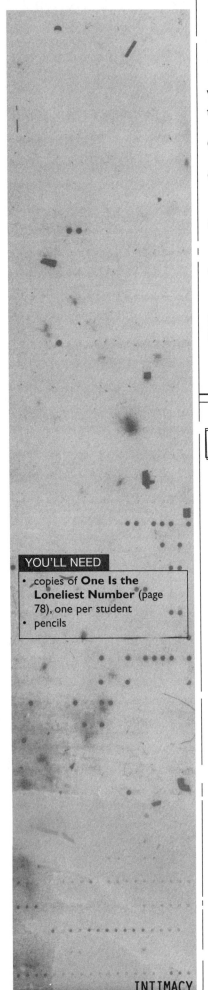

Q: Do you believe dating is the best way to find your soul mate?

Q: If you had just one minute to summarize, what advice could you give us today about dating?

When the adults are no longer in the room, follow up with these discussion questions.

Q: What do you respect about that couple's love relationship? Why?

Q: Do you think anything they shared about dating and a relationship is still relevant today? What is no longer relevant?

Q: Why does it seem so hard to find really good examples of loving intimate relationships that have lasted a long time?

Q: What are some things that we can do right now to make sure that our relationships remain intimate and long lasting?

For even more follow-up, use the material found in **Love Stories** (page 77 in this book) for group discussion or individual reflection.

word from God

— Bible study —
ONE IS THE LONELIEST NUMBER

Recognizing—and hopefully avoiding—some red flags in an intimate dating relationship.

Way before the *Guinness Book of World Records*, there lived the strongest man who ever walked the earth. His name was Samson, and he lived under a Nazirite vow (Judges 13:7, 16:17), which was a special pledge in the Old Testament that had four conditions:
1. **He could not have wine or any product of a grape vine.**
2. **He could not cut his hair or beard.**
3. **He could not touch a dead body.**
4. **He could not eat food that was designated as unclean by Jewish dietary laws.**

By keeping these four obligations, a Nazirite was designated for some special kind of service, which in Samson's case meant Herculean physical strength.

Ask for a male and female student to help you read Judges 16:4-22. The male student can read Samson's lines and the female can read Delilah's lines. You can play the part of the narrator. Explain that although Samson was an Israelite, he seemed to have a fascination with foreign women, including a Philistine woman he almost married in Judges 14 and Delilah whom we meet in Judges 16.

Q: What words would you use to describe Delilah?

Q: How would you describe her effect on Samson and his vow to God?
  • Go back and look at verses 1 to 3. Given what's there, how much blame do you believe Delilah deserves compared to, I don't know—Samson!?
  • I don't really have a follow-up question, I just want to take a moment to think about the weird fact that God sometimes works through idiots like Samson—and me.

YOU'LL NEED
• copies of **One Is the Loneliest Number** (page 78), one per student
• pencils

Q: Imagine that after the first or second time Delilah tried to find out the secret to Samson's strength, he told you and some other friends what was happening with her. What advice would you have given him?
- Do you believe if Samson had you for a friend, this story might have turned out differently? Why?
- If one of your friends expressed concern about the quality of your current relationship, how do you think you would feel? Why?

Divide the room in half. Ask students on one side of the room to share an idea about how a dating relationship can help a person's relationship with God. Then, those on the other side of the room can share an idea of how dating can hurt a person's relationship with God. Continue going back and forth several times, eventually inviting students from both sides to contribute to both topics.

Q: What's the best way you've heard in this group that a dating relationship can help your relationship with God? Why did that impress you?
- What about ways dating can threaten your relationship with God? Talk about that.

Q: Are you familiar with the idea of group dating (several couples and individuals doing things together)?
- Have you had any experience, positive or negative, with group dating?
- How do you think group dating might contribute to what we've been talking about?
- What do you think you might have to gain or lose by group dating? Because—

To help students reflect even further on implications for their own lives from the story of Samson and Delilah, use **One Is the Loneliest Number** (page 78 in this book) for additional personal or group discussion.

~~the~~ ~~last~~ word

= Bible-driven discussion =
THE YOKE'S ON YOU

The costs and benefits of intimate relationships.

Read 2 Corinthians 6:14-18.

Q: What stands out to you in these verses? Why do you think that's significant?

When Paul uses the image of being unequally yoked, he's actually referring to two farm animals in a double harness who are so incompatible they can't possibly pull together (see Deuteronomy 22:10). The name Belial, in verse 15, comes from Jewish literature. Belial refers to a personalized force opposed to God.

Ask students to move to the place in the room that most nearly reflects where they stand on each statement. The far end of the room means they disagree completely. The middle means they're not sure where they stand. The near end of the room means they agree completely. Go left to right if it works better in your space. Tell them you'll read the statement, then you'll say *Go*.

When they arrive at their position on each statement, invite them to get a partner and take 30 seconds each to tell why they're standing where they are. Time them as accurately as you wish.
- I have been incompatibly yoked with an unbeliever (or with a believer if you consider yourself an unbeliever).

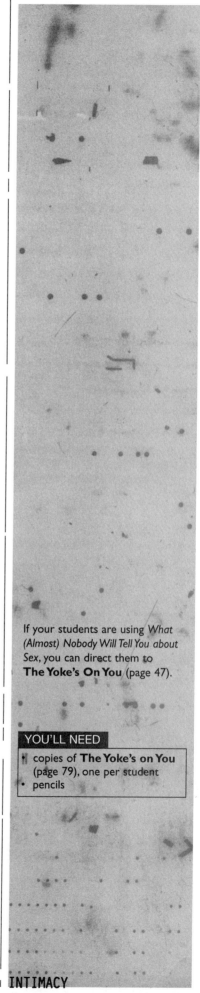

If your students are using *What (Almost) Nobody Will Tell You about Sex,* you can direct them to **The Yoke's On You** (page 47).

YOU'LL NEED
- copies of **The Yoke's on You** (page 79), one per student
- pencils

- I am presently incompatibly yoked with an unbeliever (or with a believer if you consider yourself an unbeliever).
- I have been yoked with an unbeliever (or with a believer if you think of yourself as an unbeliever) but I never thought we were incompatible.
- I am presently yoked with an unbeliever (or with a believer if you consider yourself an unbeliever), but I don't think we are incompatible.
- I believe it would be incompatible to go into business with someone who doesn't believe essentially the same things about God as I do.
- I don't see any problem with marrying someone whose beliefs are totally opposite from mine.
- Dating an unbeliever (or a believer) makes me nervous because, sooner or later, I know we'll clash on something important and one of us will have to compromise to hold on to the relationship.
- My belief in Jesus creates misunderstandings between me and my unbelieving friends (or vice versa).
- My most intimate friends don't share many of my most deeply held beliefs and values.

Invite everyone to sit down and think through some questions together.

Q: Were there any uncomfortable moments for you in this process? Why is that?

Q: Were there any surprises? Talk about that.

Q: Have you ever seen a Christian in an incompatible yoke with an unbeliever? Or a Christian trying to maintain an intimate association with someone who actively opposed God? If so, what did that look like to you?
  • What happened between them in the long run?
  • What did you learn from that? How much like Paul's words did that look like to you?

Q: What arguments have you heard on why it's wrong for believers and unbelievers to date?

Q: What arguments have you heard on why it is okay for believers and unbelievers to date?

Q: Bottom line: How do you feel about believers and unbelievers going out? Why?

Q: Read 1 Corinthians 9:19-23. How do you think these lines relate to 2 Corinthians 6:14-16? (Read those verses now.)
  • Do you think Paul is contradicting himself in these two passages? Why?

One possibility is that he's talking about two different kinds of relationships. In 1 Corinthians 9 Paul is talking about his work as an apostle. In 2 Corinthians 6 he seems to be talking about essential lifestyle links between believers and nonbelievers.

Q: The image of our bodies as temples of the Holy Spirit is fairly common among Christians. What does Paul seem to think that means in this passage?
  • How easy is that for you to accept?

I BUY IT 100%	I'M A BIT CONFUSED	I FIND IT HARD TO ACCEPT

  • Talk about the reason for your answer.

For additional discussion questions or individual reflection ideas to conclude this lesson, see **The Yoke's on You** (page 79 in this book).

In other words

PERFECT PARTNER | VIDEO

Is there a perfect dating partner? How about an almost perfect dating partner? Either way, what would make them perfect?

After you play the "**Perfect Partner**" segment, lead the following discussion.

Q: What external qualities are you looking for in a partner?
• How about internal qualities?

Q: Several people on the video mentioned things they found physically attractive in a partner. How important do you believe physical attraction is in a healthy dating relationship?
• Money was also a big theme, especially for the girls as they thought about their ideal guy. How do you feel about that?

Q: How similar, or how different, do you think girls' images of a perfect guy are from guys' images of a perfect girl?

Q: Does the perfect person even exist?

Q: Your friend says, "All of a sudden I'm seeing my boyfriend's flaws." What would you tell your friend?

YOU'LL NEED

• TV or video projection unit
• VCR or DVD player
• *Good Sex* video cued to **"Perfect Partner"** [4:55]

another video discussion starter

WILL YOU GO OUT WITH ME? | VIDEO

Everyone feels a little nervous about asking someone out or being asked out.

We're not endorsing everything in this movie, we're just saying this clip is useful. If that makes you or your boss uncomfortable, let your conscience be your guide.

Show the 45-second scene that depicts the awkwardness of a male character asking a girl out.

Q: Guys, how does this scene reflect how you feel when you are getting ready to ask out a girl?

Q: Do you ask girls out as frequently as you'd like? Why is that?

Q: Girls, what would you like guys to know about how you want to be asked out?

Q: Do you wish girls had more or less freedom to ask boys out? Why?

To help students think more about their own feelings and experiences in being asked out, or doing the asking, use the material included on **Will You Go Out with Me?** (page 80 in this book) in large or small group discussion, or as a tool for personal reflection.

YOU'LL NEED

• copy of the movie *Pleasantville*, cued to the clip that begins two minutes take from the New Line Cinema logo. It begins with, "Hi. I mean hi." and ends with, "So just give me a call. Let me know."
• television or video projection unit
• VCR or DVD player
• copies of **Will You Go Out with Me?** (page 80), one per student
• pencils

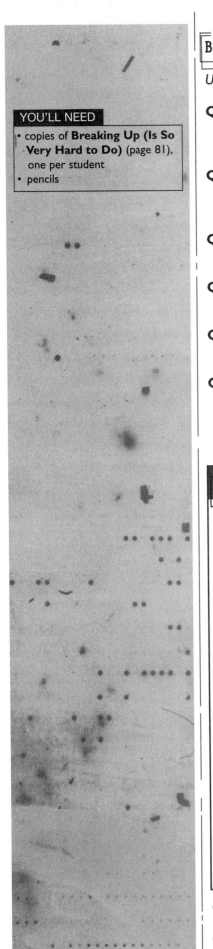

BREAKING UP (IS SO VERY HARD TO DO)

Understanding and coping with the grief involved in breaking up.

Q: Without naming names, describe the messiest breakup you've ever seen.
  • Why do you think things went so badly?
  • What did you learn from that breakup?

Q: Describe the nicest, cleanest, most godly breakup you've ever seen.
  • What factors do you think made that less painful than other breakups?
  • What did you learn from that break up?

Q: If you have been involved in a breakup, how long did it take you to get over the relationship? (Or how long do you think it will take?)

Q: Looking back over that time, was it worth it all in the end? Is it better to love and lose than to never love at all?

Q: Did you get through the pain in one step or did you experience waves of regret and loss and loneliness?

Q: Many people report going more or less nuts after a breakup. Have you seen friends react to a breakup in any of these ways? Talk about what you think was behind the behaviors you've observed.

YOU'LL NEED
- copies of **Breaking Up (Is So Very Hard to Do)** (page 81), one per student
- pencils

A = ALWAYS	S = SOMETIMES	N = ALMOST NEVER

A S N	Gaining weight
A S N	Heavy drinking
A S N	Rebounding into an unhealthy relationship
A S N	Feeling suicidal
A S N	Losing weight
A S N	Nail biting
A S N	Fighting
A S N	Having trouble sleeping
A S N	Sleeping too much
A S N	Having sexual compulsions
A S N	Having trouble concentrating
A S N	Dropping in performance at school
A S N	Having outbursts of anger
A S N	Becoming isolated from others
A S N	Refusing ever to be alone, surrounding themselves with others

Q: What did it take for your friends to come out on the other side?

Q: Were you able to contribute to their recovery? Talk about that.

To help students think even further about what they themselves have experienced when an intimate relationship dissolved, use the questions found on **Breaking Up (Is So Very Hard to Do)** (page 81 in this book) for additional large or small group discussion, or as a tool for personal reflection.

list-making activity
ONE-ANOTHERING

Intimate relationships in the context of the one-another passages in Scripture.

I'm going to read some of the passages in the Bible that use the term *one another* or something really close to it. There are lots more than just these, but we'd be here all day if we read them all. After each one, I want you to identify the command, and we'll write it on this list.

Do not steal. Do not lie. Do not deceive one another. (Leviticus 19:11)

Administer true justice; show mercy and compassion to one another. (Zechariah 7:9)

Salt is good, but if it loses its saltiness, how can you make it salty again? Have salt in yourselves, and be at peace with each other. (Mark 9:50)

A new command I give you: Love one another. As I have loved you, so you must love one another. (John 13:34)

Be devoted to one another in brotherly love. Honor one another above yourselves. (Romans 12:10)

Live in harmony with one another. Do not be proud, but be willing to associate with people of low position. Do not be conceited. (Romans 12:16)

Accept one another, then, just as Christ accepted you, in order to bring praise to God. (Romans 15:7)

I myself am convinced, my brothers, that you yourselves are full of goodness, complete in knowledge and competent to instruct one another. (Romans 15:14)

You, my brothers, were called to be free. But do not use your freedom to indulge the sinful nature; rather, serve one another in love. (Galatians 5:13)

Be completely humble and gentle; be patient, bearing with one another in love. (Ephesians 4:2)

Be kind and compassionate to one another, forgiving each other, just as in Christ God forgave you. (Ephesians 4:32)

Therefore encourage one another and build each other up, just as in fact you are doing. (1 Thessalonians 5:11)

Make sure that nobody pays back wrong for wrong, but always try to be kind to each other and to everyone else. (1 Thessalonians 5:15)

And let us consider how we may spur one another on toward love and good deeds. (Hebrews 10:24)

Therefore confess your sins to each other and pray for each other so that you may be healed. (James 5:16)

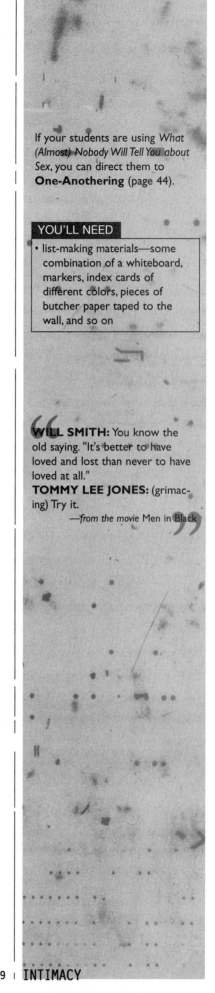

If your students are using *What (Almost) Nobody Will Tell You about Sex*, you can direct them to **One-Anothering** (page 44).

YOU'LL NEED

- list-making materials—some combination of a whiteboard, markers, index cards of different colors, pieces of butcher paper taped to the wall, and so on

WILL SMITH: You know the old saying. "It's better to have loved and lost than never to have loved at all."
TOMMY LEE JONES: (grimacing) Try it.
—*from the movie* Men in Black

Above all, love each other deeply, because love covers over a multitude of sins. 1 (Peter 4:8)

Q: What do you think is the point in all this one-anothering?

Q: Which one-another commands do you think could realistically happen in a friend-ship?

Q: Which of the one-another commands do you think could realistically happen in a dating relationship? Why?
- What could get in the way of that kind of commitment to each other?
- How would a dating relationship look different if it were bursting with examples of these one-another commands?
- Where do you think it's easier for people to *one-another*—in a friendship or dating relationship? Explain your answer.
- What are the spiritual qualities of someone who could *one-another* you back in a dating relationship or a friendship?

Q: What are some one-another ideas you think you could try this week?
- What do you need from God to carry out your plan?
- Is there someone you trust to encourage you specifically in your mission? If not, why not?

┌ Bible study ┐
FOUR LOVES

The kinds of love we share in different kinds of relationships.

> **Greek, the primary language of the New Testament, has several different words for love, four to be exact. Two of them appear prominently in the New Testament.**
>
> - *Agape* (uh-**GAH**-pay) is the unconditional love God shows us and the unconditional love we can likewise show to others (see Mark 12:31).
> - *Philia* (fill-**EE**-ah) is affectionate love for a friend (see Romans 12:10), from which we get the name Philadelphia.
> - *Eros* (**AIR**-oss) is sexual love that desires another person, from which we get the word erotic. (The word *eros* doesn't appear in the New Testament, but the idea is all over the Jewish scriptures—especially the Song of Songs.)
> - *Storge* (**STOR**-gay) is the love shared in healthy families. (This word is also absent in the New Testament, but present in spirit.)

Q: When Jesus walked on earth, do you think it was possible for him to experience or express *eros* love for someone? Why?

Read Hebrews 4:14-16 with your students.

Q: What do you think this says about Jesus and *eros*?

Q: Do you believe it's possible for us to have more than one of these kinds of love toward each other?

Q: Which kind of love do you think needs the most work in your life? Why is that?

If your students are using *What (Almost) Nobody Will Tell You about Sex*, you can direct them to **Four Loves** (page 43).

YOU'LL NEED
- copies of **Four Loves** (page 82), one per student
- pencils

For the following questions it might be best to have these four loves and their descriptions written in a place where your students can see them—projected on a wall, written on butcher paper, or given as handouts for each person.

Q: Have you seen or experienced a shift from friendly love to erotic love?
  • Do you think it turned out well or badly? Why?
  • Have you seen or experienced a shift from erotic love to friendly love?

Q: Put a percentage beside each kind of love to indicate how appropriate it is in that type of relationship. The total of all four kinds of love should be 100 percent.

FAMILY RELATIONSHIPS

_____ % unconditional love

_____ % friendly love

_____ % erotic love

_____ % family love

100 %

FRIENDSHIPS

_____ % unconditional love

_____ % friendly love

_____ % erotic love

_____ % family love

100 %

DATING

_____ % unconditional love

_____ % friendly love

_____ % erotic love

_____ % family love

100 %

MARRIAGE

_____ % unconditional love

_____ % friendly love

_____ % erotic love

_____ % family love

100 %

EVERYONE ELSE

_____ % unconditional love

_____ % friendly love

_____ % erotic love

_____ % family love

100 %

Q: If someone asked how to keep a healthy balance of the four loves in a dating relationship, what would you tell them?

To help students analyze their own balancing act with these four loves, use the questions from **Four Loves** (page 82 in this book) for subsequent group or personal reflection.

If your students are using What (Almost) Nobody Will Tell You about Sex, you can direct them to **Best Buds** (page 40).

YOU'LL NEED

- copies of **Best Buds** (page 83) one per student
- pencils

BEST BUDS

Some of the dynamics of nonsexual intimacy with friends of the same gender.

Saul was the king of Israel during a funky time. You see, David had been anointed to be the next king when he was younger, but Saul still had the top job.

As a result, Saul was insanely jealous of David and all the successes he was having in war and in winning the affection of the people. In a fit of rage, Saul tried to kill David, but because David was God's chosen, he was just fine, thank you very much.

To add insult to Saul's injured ego, David established an incredible relationship with Saul's son, Jonathan, that the Bible describes as being something very special. It even says that David loved Jonathan as himself. That's a lot of lovin'.

Read with your students the plan that David and Jonathan, David's best friend and Saul's son, put into action in 1 Samuel 20:1-42. Then use the following questions for discussion.

Q: Do you think David and Jonathan experienced true intimacy as friends? Why do you think this?

Q: Do you think friendship with someone of the same gender is inherently different than friendship with someone of the opposite gender?

Q: Do you think it's okay to only have friends of the same gender? Why?

Q: Do you think it's okay to only have friends of the opposite gender?

Q: Over the years, a few people have suggested David and Jonathan must have been homosexual lovers. What do you think about that? Why?

In 1 Samuel 20:12-15 Jonathan seems to recognize that David has a special calling from God and will have quite a dynasty. But as Saul's son, Jonathan is supposed to be the next king.

Q: What does Jonathan's willingness to surrender his right to be king say about his friendship with David?

Q: Do you think that very many people have that kind of intimacy? Why?

To help students reflect on their own intimacy with other friends of the same gender, use the questions included on **Best Buds** (page 83 in this book) for group or personal reflection.

If your students are using What (Almost) Nobody Will Tell You about Sex, you can direct them to **To Wed or Not to Wed** (page 48).

YOU'LL NEED

- copies of **To Wed or Not to Wed** (page 84), one per student
- pencils

TO WED OR NOT TO WED

The pluses and minuses of remaining single.

Here's some background—

The church in Corinth was pretty messed up. As a matter of fact, the whole of Corinth was pretty messed up. Even among the pagan world, this city had a reputation as being the worst of the worst— that says a lot in itself.

Some of the church leaders wrote Paul a letter asking his advice about some things that they were a little confused about. However, it took Paul about seven chapters to get around to answering their

questions. **He begins chapter 7 with, "Now for the matters you wrote about..."**

Read 1 Corinthians 7:25-40 with your students and then use the following questions for discussion.

Q: After reading 1 Corinthians 7:25-40, do you believe Paul is promarriage, anti-marriage, or neutral?

Q: Do you think Paul is speaking here to Christians everywhere and in all circumstances or specifically to the Christian folk at Corinth? What verses can you use to support your answer?

Q: According to this passage, how are married people different from single people?

Q: Is being single better than being married? Why or why not?

Q: Do you think there are advantages to being married that Paul doesn't mention?

Q: Do you think there are advantages to being single that Paul doesn't mention?

Q: Do you believe it's possible to be married and still serve God wholeheartedly? Why?

Q: Do you believe it's possible to be single your whole life and still feel good about yourself? Given how Paul felt about singleness, why do you think we even have to ask the question today?

To help students apply Paul's principles to their own lives, use the questions in **To Wed or Not to Wed** (page 84 in this book) for additional large group discussion, small group conversation, or as a tool for individual, personal reflection.

┌─ debate ─────────────────────────────
│ THEY KISSED DATING GOODBYE │
└──────────────────────────────────────

A debate identifying the pros and cons of dating relationships.

Pick up to six of your most opinionated and expressive students and ask them to come to the front of your room. Divide them into two teams, and hand each team a piece of paper. You might want to give each team three to five minutes to come up with some arguments that support its own position.

On one piece of paper write, BE PREPARED TO DEBATE THIS VIGOROUSLY EVEN IF YOU DON'T BELIEVE IT: CHRISTIANS SHOULD NEVER DATE EACH OTHER. THERE SHOULD NOT BE ANY PHYSICAL EXPRESSION OF LOVE BEFORE A COUPLE IS MARRIED.

On another piece of paper write, BE PREPARED TO DEBATE THIS VIGOROUSLY EVEN IF YOU DON'T BELIEVE IT: IT IS FINE FOR CHRISTIANS TO DATE EACH OTHER. PHYSICAL EXPRESSION OF INTIMACY IS A PERFECTLY NORMAL WAY FOR TWO PEOPLE TO SHOW AFFECTION. KISSING DATING GOODBYE IS RIDICULOUS!

Some people believe there's no room for erotic expression of any kind before people are married. In other words, they believe you shouldn't date in the contemporary sense before you are committed to marry someone. In this scenario you'd remain friends with someone, getting to know them better and better—but you wouldn't date or get involved physically with them. On the other side of this argument, some people believe that dating is the best way for a couple to prepare for marriage and a lifetime commitment to each other. Here to debate this issue are...

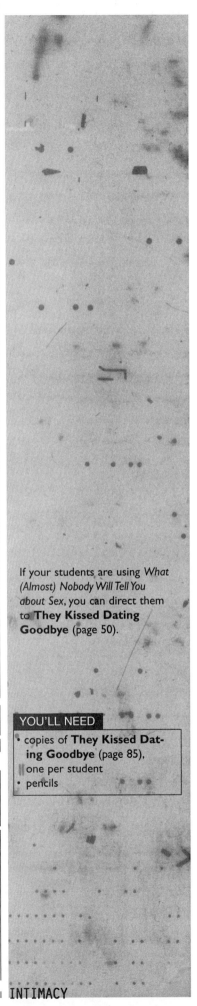

If your students are using *What (Almost) Nobody Will Tell You about Sex*, you can direct them to **They Kissed Dating Goodbye** (page 50).

YOU'LL NEED

• copies of **They Kissed Dating Goodbye** (page 85), one per student
• pencils

After the smoke clears—

Q: How would you summarize the points of view presented here?

Q: Was anything brought up here that challenged the way you think about dating?

Q: Suppose you kissed dating goodbye. What problems might that create for you?

Q: Suppose you choose to go out in a typical pattern of dating from now on. What problems might that create for you?

Q: Would dating like everybody else solve any problems for you?

Q: How compatible do you think American-style dating is with Christianity?

Completely compatible, because—

Needs work, but still compatible because—

Completely incompatible, because—

Q: What could make it more Christ-like?

Q: As a group, where do we stand on the issue? Should we just say no to dating? Why or why not?
  • If we answer that we shouldn't say no to dating, what should we make sure to avoid in a dating relationship so that we experience healthy intimacy?

To help students consider their own experience with and feelings about dating, distribute **They Kissed Dating Goodbye** (page 85 in this book) for personal reflection, or use it as material for additional large or small group discussion.

---

 evaluation activity
ROOKIE MISTAKES

Common relationship mistakes that each gender makes.

Get an adult partner of the other gender to help you lead this discussion of common mistakes people make in relationships. Consider dividing the room in two and putting guys on one side and girls on the other—just to see what happens.

When it comes to dating, everybody makes rookie mistakes, right? We're going to take a look at some common errors and see what we can do to help each other learn from our mistakes.

Distribute copies of **Mistakes Girls Make** (page 86) to everyone. Review its ideas one at a time, inviting students of either gender to agree, disagree, share experiences, or comment on each item.

When you're finished, lead the following discussion:

Q: If someone asked what you think causes the mistakes some girls make with guys, what would you tell them?

Q: When, if ever, do you think girls stop making these mistakes?

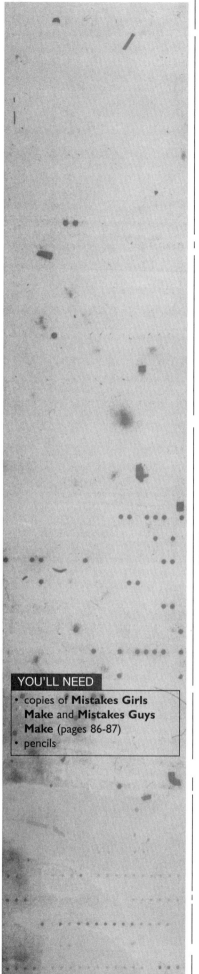

YOU'LL NEED
• copies of **Mistakes Girls Make** and **Mistakes Guys Make** (pages 86-87)
• pencils

Now, go over **Mistakes Guys Make** (page 87 in this book) with your students and answer the following questions together:

Q: If someone asked what you think causes the mistakes some guys make with girls, what would you tell them?

Q: When, if ever, do you think guys stop making these mistakes?

Q: Do you think these mistakes are any less likely to happen between two Christians than two unbelievers?

Q: Given these mistakes, what changes have you realized you need to make?

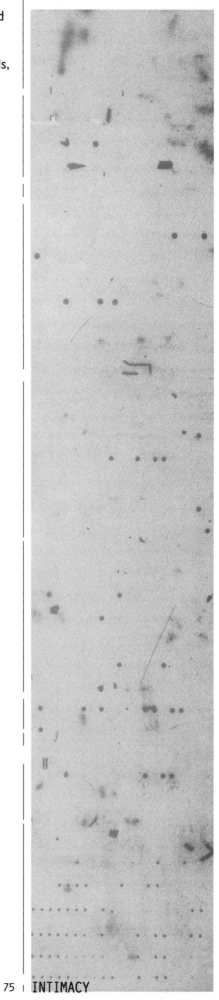

INTIMACY

Q: Did you feel uncomfortable about anyone or anything that was in the video? Why?
  • What, if anything, did you agree with?

Q: Have you made mistakes with intimacy? Write about that.
  • If so, what did you find out about yourself?
  • What did you find out about someone else?
  • What did you find out about intimacy?

Q: When you think about intimacy, which attitudes and emotions apply?
  ☐ Anticipation because...

  ☐ Fear because...

  ☐ Regret because...

  ☐ Hope because...

Q: What do you think you still have to learn about intimacy?
  • From whom do you think you might get help?
  • How do you think you could ask for that help?

LOVE STORIES

Q: Do you remember the interview that you saw in your group with the older couple who had been together for a while? How does this make you feel about your own future dating life?

Q: What do you respect about their love relationship? Why?

Q: What do you think you would have to do to get what they have?

Q: How do you think these love stories compare to the relationship between your parents?

Q: If you marry, how do you think your relationship with your spouse will be different from your parents' relationship? Why?

Q: Are there any fresh commitments you need to make about your dating life?

ONE IS THE LONELIEST NUMBER

Reflect on these questions by yourself or with your group.

Q: If you are dating someone now, what do you think your closest friends would say about that person?
- Have you asked your friends' opinions about him or her? Why is that?

Q: If you are dating someone now, how do you think your closest friends would say this person is affecting your relationship with God?
- Have you asked your friends' opinions about that person's influence on your relationship with God? Why is that?
- If you were your own best friend, what would you say about the spiritual influence of the person you're dating?
- What would you say about your spiritual influence on the person you're going out with?

Q: Think about one of your close friendships for a moment. How does that relationship affect your relationship with God?

Q: Can you think of one thing you could do in a dating relationship or friendship that would help you both grow closer to God?
- What would you have to gain by that?
- Would you have anything to lose?

THE YOKE'S ON YOU

Q: What's the difference between close friendship and being yoked together with another person?
- If you wanted to lead someone to faith in Jesus, are you prepared to be that person's intimate friend? Write about that.
- Do you think an unequal yoke could make it difficult for you to lead another person to faith in Christ?

Q: Have you been unequally yoked with another person? If so, write a brief outline of the beginning, middle, and end of that story.

Being unequally yoked started when—

I realized I was unequally yoked when—

Things changed when—

Q: Have you ever been influenced by a friend in a way that you regretted later? Write about that. Have you ever been influenced by a friend in a way that you later appreciated? Write about that.

Q: If someone asked you to describe the friends who have made a positive difference in your life, what would you say about them? How does this description compare to—
- people you've gone out with in the past?
- the person you're going out with now?
- the kind of person you'd like to go out with?
- the kind of person you want to become?

Q: Have you ever influenced a friend in a way they later appreciated? Have you influenced a friend in a way they later regretted? Write about what happened.

Q: If you can think of an area where you'd like to grow into a better friend, write a brief plan to help you get from where you are now to where you'd like to be—including getting support to help you grow.

WILL
YOU
GO
OU
WIT
ME

WILL YOU GO OUT WITH ME?

Use these questions to reflect by yourself or with your group.

Q: If you're a girl, do you feel comfortable asking a guy out?

Q: If you're a guy, how would you feel if a girl asked you out?

Q: What scares you about asking someone out?

Q: Does anything scare you about being asked out?

Q: Have you ever accepted a date because you didn't know how to decline the invitation?
- If so, why was it hard to decline?
- How did things turn out?
- Did you learn anything useful from the experience?

Q: What do you think is the best way to ask someone out?

Q: What is the best way to decline a date?

BREAKING UP (IS SO VERY HARD TO DO)

Answer the questions below.

Q: What do you think it takes for a breakup to go well?
- What do you think is the biggest barrier to that?

Q: If you've gone through a breakup, how painful was it compared to the greatest emotional pain you ever had?

- Let's say the greatest pain you ever endured was a 10. Now circle the number that describes your breakup.

1   2   3   4   5   6   7   8   9   10

Q: Did you go a little nuts after your breakup? Circle and talk about all the following that apply to you.

- I gained weight.
- I drank heavily.
- I rebounded into an unhealthy relationship.
- I felt suicidal.
- I lost weight.
- I started biting my nails.
- I got into fights.
- I had trouble sleeping.

- I slept too much.
- I was sexually compulsive.
- I had trouble concentrating.
- I had trouble with my grades at school.
- I had angry blowups.
- I isolated myself from others.
- I hated being alone, so I constantly surrounded myself with people.

Q: What did it take for you to come out on the other side?
- How long did that take?
- Who contributed to your recovery?
- Where do you think God was in all that? How did that make you feel?

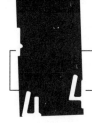

FOUR LOVES

FOUR LOVES

Reflect on these questions by yourself or with your group.

In Greek, the primary language of the New Testament, there are several different words for love—four, to be exact. Two of them appear prominently in the New Testament.

- *Agape* (uh-GAH-pay) is the unconditional love God shows us and the unconditional love we can likewise show to others (see I John 4:7).
- *Philia* (fill-EE-ah) is affectionate love for a friend (see Romans 12:10), from which we get the name Philadelphia.
- *Eros* (AIR-oss) is sexual love that desires another person, from which we get the word *erotic*. (The word *eros* doesn't appear in the New Testament, but the idea is all over the Jewish scriptures—especially the Song of Songs.)
- *Storge* (STOR-gay) is the love shared in healthy families. (This word is also absent in the New Testament, but present in spirit.)

Q: Think back a year and compare where you were then with where you are now in each of the four loves.

- Family love
    - ☐ Worse then because...
    - ☐ About the same because...
    - ☐ Better because...

- Friendly love
    - ☐ Worse then because...
    - ☐ About the same because...
    - ☐ Better because...

- Erotic love
    - ☐ Worse then because...
    - ☐ About the same because...
    - ☐ Better because...

- Unconditional love
    - ☐ Worse then because...
    - ☐ About the same because...
    - ☐ Better because...

Q: Given what you've just written, are there things you'd like to do differently to help those areas where you're a little worse than you were last year?

DEAR GOD, Write a prayer of thanksgiving and hope. Thank God for where you're better (or no worse) off. Ask God to help you make the progress you need to make to be where you'd like to be this time next year.

www.YouthSpecialties.cc[...]

BEST BUDS

Q: Who are your closest friends?
- What makes them your closest friends?

Q: Think for a moment about what has happened in your friendships in the last year. When has intimacy been easier?

| when good things happen to me | it doesn't matter | when bad things happen to me |

- Compare that to how Jonathan seemed to feel about David eventually becoming king instead of himself. How do you feel about the comparison?

Compare 1 Samuel 20 with 1 Corinthians 13:4-7.

Q: How do you think Jonathan and David stack up in the comparison?
- Compare your closest friendships with 1 Corinthians 13:4-7. How do you think yours stack up?
- Do you see anything you could use some help with? Is there someone you know who may be able to help you?

TO WED OR NOT TO WED

Reflect on the following questions and answer.

Q: Which benefits of singleness are most appealing to you? What makes them attractive?

Q: What seem like the downsides of being single?

Q: How has your own relationship with God been different when you were dating someone than when you were not dating someone?

Q: If you could plan out your life, would you want to remain single until you're 21, 25, or 30, or even stay that way forever? Why?

• Have you seriously considered remaining single for your whole life? Talk about that.

Q: Do you have any sense about what God may have in mind for you as a married person or a single person?

Reflect on these questions.

Q: On a scale of one to 10, how would you rate your experience with dating so far?

1   2   3   4   5   6   7   8   9   10

• What do you think would make going out a better experience for you?

Q: If someone asked you to explain why you date the way you do (or why you don't date), what would you tell them?

Q: If you're going out, are you going out the way you know God wants you to?
   • If you're going out but you're not happy with the patterns you're in, what do you think would make that better?

Q: Who could you trust to tell the truth to about your dating experience?

BYE BYE

MISTAKES GIRLS MAKE

Circle the answers that apply to you.

This is a list of mistakes some girls make when they relate to guys. Do you see these mistakes—

A ALL THE TIME
S SOMETIMES
N ALMOST NEVER

When a girl is lonely or insecure—

A S N   She often doesn't really choose, she just goes out with whoever is available.

A S N   She throws herself at guys to get attention.

A S N   She works at making herself unattractive to lessen the pain.

When a girl likes a guy—

A S N   She nags the guy's friends to see if he might like her back.

A S N   She flirts, and if he doesn't notice, she flirts even harder.

A S N   She plays it cool and aloof, hoping that the guy will notice how cool she is.

When a girl starts dating a guy—

A S N   She's too busy making sure he wants her to question whether or not she wants him.

A S N   She expects him to be a knight in shining armor who will rescue her from all bad things and protect her from all harm.

A S N   She thinks he will stop behavior that bugs her.

A S N   She believes she can change him.

A S N   She lets him be her life instead of a part of her life.

A S N   Her fear of abandonment makes her clingy.

A S N   She gives physical gratification to get relational gratification.

A S N   She cuts herself off from her family.

A S N   She cuts herself off from her friends.

When a girl goes through a breakup—

A S N   Instead of taking some time apart to recover, she still tries to spend time with him as friends and keeps opening old wounds and repeating old mistakes.

Adapted from Ten Stupid Things Women Do to Mess Up Their Lives, *by Dr. Laura Schlessinger (HarperCollins).*

MISTAKES GUYS MAKE

Circle the answers that apply to you.

This is a list of mistakes some guys make when they relate to girls. Do you see these mistakes—

A ALL THE TIME
S SOMETIMES
N ALMOST NEVER

When a guy is lonely or insecure—

A S N   He gets obnoxious around girls, because he tries too hard.

A S N   He acts pitiful, hoping a girl will feel sorry for him.

When a guy likes a girl—

A S N   He lets how she looks blind him from seeing who she really is.

A S N   He shows off, usually in macho ways, trying to impress her.

A S N   He is hyperattentive, acting like she's the only person on earth.

When a guy starts dating a girl—

A S N   He tries to be a knight in shining armor who will rescue the helpless damsel from all bad things and protect her from all harm.

A S N   His girlfriend becomes a badge of honor instead of a real person.

A S N   He seeks physical gratification before relational gratification.

A S N   He lets her take care of him, more like a mother than a girlfriend.

A S N   He tries to control her and make decisions for her.

A S N   He confuses being macho with courage.

A S N   He continues in the relationship without ever evaluating its quality.

A S N   He tells her what he thinks she wants to hear in order to get sex from her.

A S N   He cuts himself off from his family.

A S N   He cuts himself off from his friends.

When a guys goes through a breakup—

A S N   He doesn't get advice from people who could help.

A S N   He walks out too quickly.

A S N   He tries to hold on too long.

A S N   He gets depressed or angry and takes it out on himself or others.

Adapted from Ten Stupid Things Men Do to Mess Up Their Lives, *by Dr. Laura Schlessinger (HarperCollins).*

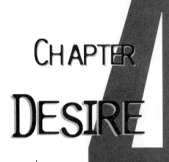

CHAPTER
DESIRE 4

before you
teach this lesson...

Desire is good. Except when it's bad.

Think about it. Desire drives one person to sacrifice herself in pursuit of a cure for AIDS. Desire drives another person to indulge in behavior that spreads HIV.

Desire is tricky that way.

Healthy desire generates commitment and propels accomplishment. Unhealthy desire, on the other hand—there's always that dreaded other hand—fuels lust. And lust, as the book of James says, gives birth to sin which, when it's full-grown, gives birth to death (James 1:15). Yikes!

Helping adolescents cultivate healthy desires and avoid being seduced by unhealthy desires is what this chapter is about. It's no secret that it's not as easy as it sounds.

Desire is so easily twisted:
I like it becomes *I want it.*
I want it becomes *I need it.*
I need it becomes *You owe it to me.*
Which becomes *Never mind, I'll just take it.*

People get out of control when they get upside down with desire. And maybe that's what unhealthy desire is really about: we seize control when we don't get what we want exactly when we want it.

Stupid? You bet. Unusually stupid? Not in the least. Everyone falls under the spell of unhealthy desire at some point.

- A tenth grader with an appetite for fine dining finds himself craving far too much of a good thing because his mood elevates when he eats and falls when he's hungry.
- A senior, who likes a tidy room, becomes so obsessed with neatness that no one comes to his house anymore—which is fine since people are such slobs anyway.
- A ninth grader, who started out enjoying physical pleasure as much as the next person, takes a wrong turn into sexual compulsion and doesn't even know how it happened, let alone how to get back to the main road.

Food, tidiness, pleasure—it's all good. But, when desire turns bottom side up, beautiful things turn ugly. It's not hard to see what unhealthy desire does to relationships. The people we deal with are young and inexperienced, no matter how mature or sophisticated they may appear. Look for telltale signs.

- Kids get selfish and pushy when the one thing they desire is the very thing or experience or relationship they can't have. Watch for aggressive or obnoxious behavior—not belligerent, necessarily, but disagreeable nonetheless.
- Those who feel they're entitled to more than they're getting start taking more than they give. Watch for foot-dragging, tardiness, incomplete follow-through, testing limits, whining, and other passive resistance. Listen for reports from their friends of loyalty tests, tongue-lashings, and ultimatum tirades.
- When kids feel something is being withheld from them, they get sneaky and secretive. Look for lying, cover-ups, and burning bridges.

Desire is longing for something—often so much that you're driven to get it even if you have to sacrifice something else that's valuable.

I've never really been mad at God—God just has the job I want.

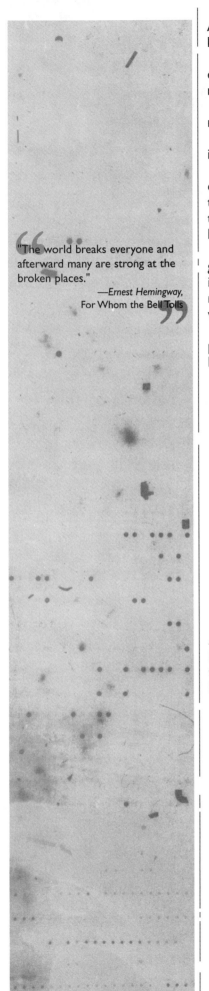

And look for someone on the other side of the relationship who says (sooner than later, we hope), "Who needs that? I'm outta here."

This is a critical moment. The young man or woman with the courage to withdraw from the one whose desire is out of control needs support and encouragement. That person's commitment to health will almost certainly be tested.

The one struggling with unhealthy desire also needs care. Because the next stop may be isolation, followed by obsession, then perversion.

If that person is male, he is more likely to take his own life than at any other time in adolescence. So try not to leave him high and dry.

In any event, look for signs of withdrawal, isolation, substance abuse, violence, and other high-risk behavior. Use your network to draw that person out. Initiate an opportunity to vent feelings without giving false hopes of rekindling the flame. Remember, they were playing with fire to begin with. If you detect signs of obsession—telephone hang-ups, stalking, self-mutilation—consider a referral to a counselor.

The apostle Paul told his flock in Corinth that God used something—he didn't give details—to keep him from being conceited. Paul says he pleaded with God to take it away again and again, but God said, "My grace is sufficient for you, for my power is made perfect in weakness" (2 Corinthians 12:9). So, Paul said, he came to delight in weakness. He's in a fairly small club—because of his delight, not his weakness.

Some interpretations hold that Paul was referring to some physical weakness, like progressive blindness, and maybe that's the case. But lay this passage next to his lament in Romans 7 and see what you get.

I know that nothing good lives in me, that is, in my sinful nature. For I have the desire to do what is good, but I cannot carry it out. For what I do is not the good I want to do; no, the evil I do not want to do—this I keep on doing. Now if I do what I do not want to do, it is no longer I who do it, but it is sin living in me that does it. So I find this law at work: When I want to do good, evil is right there with me. For in my inner being I delight in God's law; but I see another law at work in the members of my body, waging war against the law of my mind and making me a prisoner of the law of sin at work within my members. What a wretched man I am! Who will rescue me from this body of death? Thanks be to God—through Jesus Christ our Lord!

So then, I myself in my mind am a slave to God's law, but in the sinful nature a slave to the law of sin.

—Romans 7:18-25

Again, some interpretations explain this away; they say he was talking about life before he was a Christian. But the evidence suggests another possibility. It's possible that Paul struggled with an unhealthy desire so powerful only Jesus could overcome it. If that's true, Paul wasn't alone in his struggle. Because desire is tricky that way.

reflect a moment...

To help your students most effectively, you need to make every effort to process your own sexual experiences, questions, and struggles. Here are some questions to get thinking:

Q: What has been your most positive experience with healthy desire?
- Did you face the temptation to desire the right thing for the wrong reason? If so, how did you cope with that?

Q: What has been your most negative experience with unhealthy desire?
- Is that resolved? If so, how did you get resolution? If not, how would you describe your current situation?

Q: What do you think it would cost you to be open about your struggle with unhealthy desire? Do you think you can afford that risk?

Q: If you had just one hour to talk with kids about desire, what would you try to communicate?
- Why do you think that's so important?
- How would you try to communicate during that hour?

In our own words

video discussion starter

DESIRE ──────────────────────────────── VIDEO

Desire is often good, and sometimes bad, but rarely indifferent.

After playing the **"Desire"** segment, lead the following discussion.

Q: When is desire good?
- When is desire bad?

Q: How does desire lead to selfishness? How have you seen it lead to selfishness in others or in you?

YOU'LL NEED
- TV or video projection unit
- VCR or DVD player
- *Good Sex* video cued to **"Desire"** [24:05]

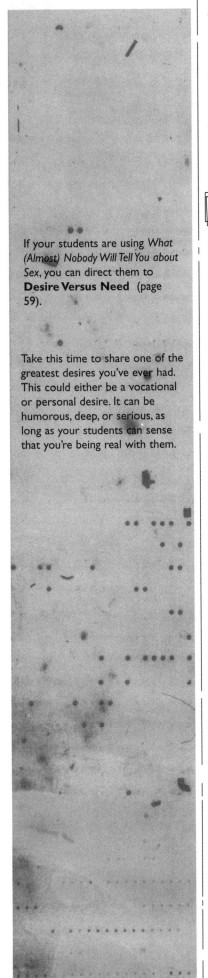

If your students are using *What (Almost) Nobody Will Tell You about Sex*, you can direct them to **Desire Versus Need** (page 59).

Take this time to share one of the greatest desires you've ever had. This could either be a vocational or personal desire. It can be humorous, deep, or serious, as long as your students can sense that you're being real with them.

Q: What do you think of this statement: *I want something so bad it hurts, but when I get it, it hurts more.* Do you believe this is true or not? Can you give any examples of your own life to support your opinion?

Q: Is it possible that God can help us control our desires?
• What about people who don't know God? Can they control their desires also?

Q: What do you think of the hope that God can change what we need into what we want? Does that seem true to you, or not?

DESIRE VERSUS NEED

A wrestling match between desire and need.

The dictionary defines *desire* as something longed for, a craving, a wish.

Q: What's the one thing you desire more than anything right now? Is it a realistic desire? How do you believe it lines up with God's plan for your life?

Q: A lot of people say that desire in and of itself is not a good or bad thing. Do you agree?

Q: Who are some people who've used desire for evil? (You can name famous people or, if you can do it without embarrassing anyone, more ordinary people.)

Q: What about some folks who've used their desires for good? (With this question, you could encourage your students not just to mention Mother Teresa, but also the name of the girl sitting next to them.)

Q: All these people we just mentioned had really strong desires. What do you think makes one person's desire cause her to destroy and another person's desire cause him to help and support?

We've already read that desire is something to long for, a craving, a wish. But this is not the only force that drives us. There is something else that we call need. The dictionary says that need is a necessity, a lack of something required. It's something we just cannot do without—If we do not get it, we die.

Q: Let's make a list of things people say they need. How many of the things that you perceive as needs really are desires?
• What are some examples of that?

Q: What about sexual desires? Do you believe sexual fulfillment is a desire or a need?

Q: How did you reach that conclusion?

Q: Is sexual desire a good or a bad thing?
• Why do you believe that?
• When can it be a good thing?
• When can it be a bad thing?

What lies beneath sexual desire—ours and others'.

Sexual desire has many faces. What can be an incredible temptation to commit sexual sin for one person could be a thing that someone else would just laugh off or find disgusting. Have a listen to a few of these stories.

BRIAN

Brian has a friend named Cory. They have been friends for years now and have spent a lot of time at each other's houses. Brian particularly loves to go to Cory's house for one reason. Cory's older sister is an unbelievable hottie. For years Brian has had sexual fantasies about his best friend's sister, but lately things have been getting worse.

Just the other day Brian had an uncontrollable urge to sneak into Cory's sister's bedroom and go through her underwear drawer. He had no idea why he was doing it, he knew that it made no sense, but something just drew him into her bedroom. Just as he was going through her underwear, Cory walked into the bedroom and caught Brain in the middle of indulging in his fantasy. Their relationship is over now, and even worse for Brian is the shame of having to go to school every day knowing that everybody knows what he was caught doing.

JACKIE

Jackie has a reputation at school. She doesn't know why she does it, but she just can't get enough. Every time she goes out with a guy on a date the desire to perform oral sex or to receive it overwhelms her. It has gotten to the point now where if at the end of a date she does not either perform this act or have it done to her, she views it as a wasted night.

She hates the way the guys never call back after that first date, and she cannot stand the way the other girls talk about her at school, but this desire has a hold on her life—she only feels complete as a sexual person when she is giving in to this sexual desire.

JOSH

Josh has been going to church with his family as long as he can remember. His mom is pretty strict. She doesn't let him see any movies rated PG-13, let alone R. She refuses to get cable for the house.

Josh doesn't mind too much, because frankly, his best friend, Austin, has cable TV —so he can watch whatever he wants to when he is over there. Plus, Austin has four movie stations, so any movie Josh missed in the theater he can just catch a few months later.

One day before the summer of their ninth-grade year, Josh and Austin were hanging out as usual, watching TV, when Austin said, "Hey, Josh, shut the door." Austin brought out some porno magazines that some of the other guys on the water polo team had given him. Josh had never seen pictures like that before, and he was intrigued. He and Austin stared at them for over a half hour. They did the same the next day, and the day after that, and the day after that.

Soon Austin even let Josh take some home with him, and Josh was careful to hide them under his mattress so his mom wouldn't find them. Whenever he had more than 10 minutes to himself in his room, he'd pull out the magazines and just stare at the beautiful and exotic women. He couldn't get enough of them.

Q: Do you know anyone who seems to be driven the way Brian, Jackie, and Josh are driven? Without embarrassing anyone or naming names, can you tell us what you know about that person's struggle?

Q: If any of them came to you seeking advice for a way to control these sexual desires, what advice would you give?

A common theme among teens is that their sexual desire is so strong they just can't stop themselves. Is it so strong that if their parents walked in on what they were doing, they still wouldn't be able to stop?

It seems Brian might be edging into fetishism. For more information on sexual fetishes, see **A Note about Sexual Fetishes** (pages 100-101 in this book).

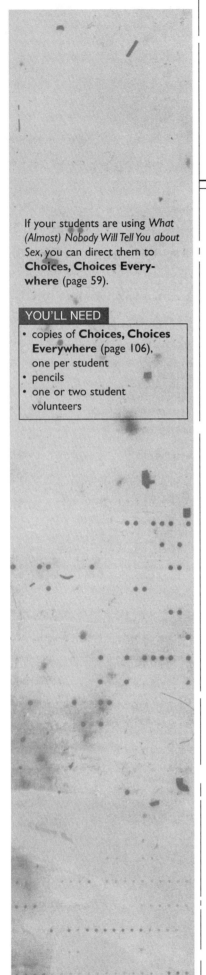

• Do you believe it's even possible for them to control their desires?

The Bible is full of stories of people who have been in similar situations as Brian, Jackie, and Josh. These people may not have wanted to go through an underwear drawer, perform oral sex, or hide porno magazines from their parents, but they were faced with situations full of equally strong sexual desire. Let's have a look at one of these times.

word from God

If your students are using *What (Almost) Nobody Will Tell You about Sex,* you can direct them to **Choices, Choices Everywhere** (page 59).

YOU'LL NEED

• copies of **Choices, Choices Everywhere** (page 106), one per student
• pencils
• one or two student volunteers

--- Bible study ---
CHOICES, CHOICES EVERYWHERE

Sexual desires come with a series of decisions.

Explain that you'd like a student or two to read 2 Samuel 11:1-17 aloud. At several places in the narrative, you're going to surprise your students by interrupting and yelling, "Stop!" The text, stop points, and questions are provided below.
The narrative begins with 2 Samuel 11:1-2.

> **In the spring, at the time when kings go off to war, David sent Joab out with the king's men and the whole Israelite army. They destroyed the Ammonites and besieged Rabbah. But David remained in Jerusalem.**
> **One evening David got up from his bed and walked around on the roof of the palace. From the roof he saw a woman bathing. The woman was very beautiful.**

Stop! Here's David, just hanging out on the roof, who knows, he may have been praying at the time, when all of a sudden he sees this hottie taking a bath.

Q: At this point has David done anything wrong?

Q: There is a theological term for what David is doing on his roof. It's called *creation appreciation.* Is it sinful to partake in creation appreciation?

Q: According to the Bible, what should David do right at this very point?

Continue with 2 Samuel 11:3.

> **And David sent someone to find out about her. The man said, "Isn't this Bathsheba, the daughter of Eliam and the wife of Uriah the Hittite?"**

Stop! Now David has just sent someone to find out who this woman was and he has discovered that this babe, who just happens to be bathing in the nude, is married.

Q: What should this piece of news have meant to King David?

Q: What options does he have at this point?

Continue with 2 Samuel 11:4-5.

> **Then David sent messengers to get her. She came to him, and he slept with her. (She had purified herself from her uncleanness.) Then she went back home. The woman conceived and sent word to David, saying, "I am pregnant."**

Stop! Okay, hold on, we go from one verse telling us that Bathsheba is married, to the next that says that David sent some of his roadies to bring her backstage.

Q: At what point in this narrative so far has David crossed the line from creation appreciation to giving in to his sexual desires? Was it—
- while he was on the roof, and he looked a little longer than he should have?
- when he sent a messenger to find out this woman's name?
- when he asked some people to send her to him?
- when he had sex with her?

There was a point in this story where David had a choice to give in to or to resist his sexual desire and fantasy. That point is long gone now. Bathsheba is pregnant, and things aren't looking good for either of them.

Q: At this point in the story, what do you think God would want David to do?

Continue with 2 Samuel 11:6-13.

> So David sent this word to Joab: "Send me Uriah the Hittite." And Joab sent him to David. When Uriah came to him, David asked him how Joab was, how the soldiers were and how the war was going. Then David said to Uriah, "Go down to your house and wash your feet" So Uriah left the palace, and a gift from the king was sent after him. But Uriah slept at the entrance to the palace with all his master's servants and did not go down to his house.
>
> When David was told, "Uriah did not go home," he asked him, "Haven't you just come from a distance? Why didn't you go home?"
>
> Uriah said to David, "The ark and Israel and Judah are staying in tents, and my master Joab and my lord's men are camped in the open fields. How could I go to my house to eat and drink and lie with my wife? As surely as you live, I will not do such a thing!"
>
> Then David said to him, "Stay here one more day, and tomorrow I will send you back." So Uriah remained in Jerusalem that day and the next. At David's invitation, he ate and drank with him, and David made him drunk. But in the evening Uriah went out to sleep on his mat among his master's servants; he did not go home.

Stop! Now David is really messed up. Uriah observed the rule that soldiers on active duty were to remain sexually abstinent. (See David's own words in 1 Samuel 21:5.) David could not even trick his faithful servant into sleeping with his wife. The hole just keeps getting deeper, and deeper, and deeper.

Q: If you were David, what would you do at this point? Would you do nothing or would you 'fess up to Uriah?

Continue with 2 Samuel 11:14-17.

> In the morning David wrote a letter to Joab and sent it with Uriah. In it he wrote, "Put Uriah in the front line where the fighting is fiercest. Then withdraw from him so he will be struck down and die."
>
> So while Joab had the city under siege, he put Uriah at a place where he knew the strongest defenders were. When the men of the city came out and fought against Joab, some

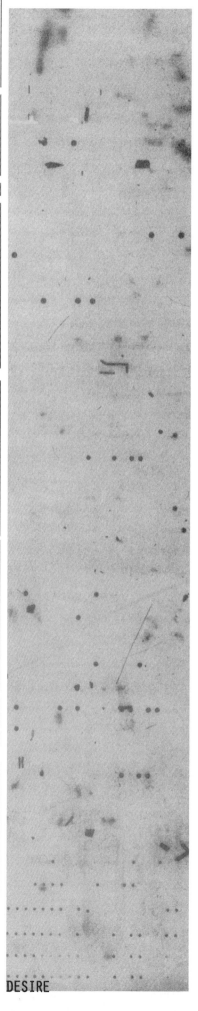

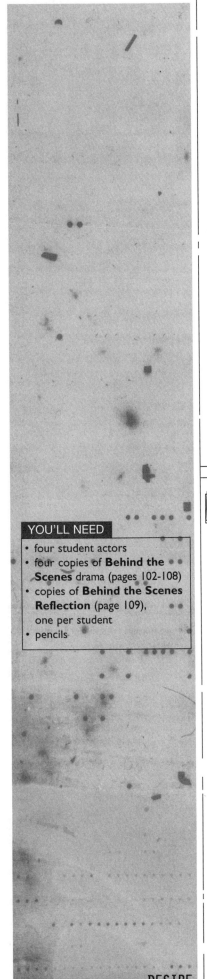

of the men in David's army fell; moreover, Uriah the Hittite was dead."

Ironically, Uriah ended up carrying his own death warrant back to battle. But it wasn't just Uriah who died because of David's act. Other men died in battle too. (See 2 Samuel 11:24.) Plus, David's cover-up wouldn't have worked well, because Bathsheba would have had to grieve for two months. So everybody would know that she had gotten pregnant before her husband was killed, but that she wasn't pregnant by him.

David eventually repented in 2 Samuel 12, but the damage had been done. At least four times he had a chance to make a good choice, be honest, and stop his sin—but he didn't.

Q: In the middle of sexual temptations and desire, how clear are our options?

Q: Why is it that even when people know the right thing to do, sometimes they choose to do the wrong thing?

Q: How does thinking about both short- and long-term consequences affect whether or not you give in to improper sexual desire? Discuss that.

To help students further process what they've learned from the story of David and Bathsheba, distribute copies of **Choices, Choices Everywhere** (page 106 in this book) and use the questions for large or small group discussion or individual, personal reflection.

the last word

drama and discussion

BEHIND THE SCENES

A behind-the-scenes look at the desires that drive what we do.

Have the students read over **Behind the Scenes** ahead of time. They don't have to memorize their lines, but they should be familiar enough with them to read through them easily. Set up four chairs—two rows of two. Lower the lights if you can to add to the mood.

As the sketch ends and the lights come back on, invite a warm round of applause for your sure-to-be-Oscar Award-winning cast and then ask the following questions:

Q: We don't know for sure what happened next for Jessica and Mario. What do you think happened? Why?

Q: Do you think people ever go through what Jessica and Mario went through? Talk about that.
  • How about you? Have you ever had that kind of experience? Can you talk about it?

Q: How are Jessica and Mario's inner voices similar?

Q: What habits and attitudes do you think lie behind Jessica and Mario's actions? I'll read a list, you tell me which ones you think fit and why.

  • Anxiety

  • Desire

  • Fear

  • Honesty

  • Hope

YOU'LL NEED
• four student actors
• four copies of **Behind the Scenes** drama (pages 102-108)
• copies of **Behind the Scenes Reflection** (page 109), one per student
• pencils

- Lust
- Old patterns
- Possessiveness
- Pride
- Self-examination
- Sneakiness.

Q: Do you believe these fears, anxieties and desires are different for people who don't call themselves Christians and people who do?

To conclude this discussion, distribute copies of **Behind the Scenes Reflections** (page 109 in this book) and ask students to individually reflect and journal about their own experiences, desires, and motivations. Encourage students to take action by talking with the person they listed in the last question about making changes.

In other words

── charade game ──
ACTING ON IMPULSE

Students consider whether sexual desires can be controlled.

Form two teams and ask for two volunteers from each team. Give the volunteer from the first team three cards from the **Acting on Impulse Game** and 30 seconds to prepare.

On each of the three cards are two desires with different numerical values corresponding to the perceived degree of difficulty—get the hard word, get more points. The first player may choose any of the six desires to act out for his team. He will have two minutes total. When his team guesses a desire correctly, he may act out additional desires for as long as time remains.

Then the volunteer from the second team gets her turn. You can alternate between the teams for as long as it's fun, or until you think you've made your point.

If you have more than 40 students, you may want to have additional teams play each other simultaneously.

Q: Which of the items was hardest for you to resist?
- Why was it hard for you to resist?

Q: It's often thought that behind every desire lies a deeper emotion. In other words, behind a craving for ice cream might lie a desire to escape some sort of pain—if only for one bowl. Behind a desire to be popular may be the fear of being left out or alone. Do you agree that there are often deeper desires behind our immediate desires?
- How do you think that relates to what might be behind our sexual desires?

For additional questions to follow up on this game, see **Acting on Impulse** (page 112 in this book) for ideas for large or small group discussion or individual reflection.

── discussion-based activity ──
GUESS WHO'S SEXUALLY ACTIVE

Surprise, surprise, we're all sexually active.

It has recently come to my attention that several members of this group are sexually active. I don't want to freak anybody out, but I've decided to name them in public right now.

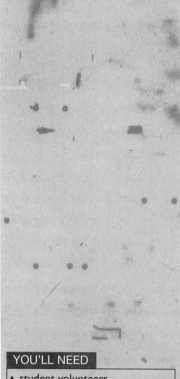

YOU'LL NEED
- student volunteers
- a stopwatch
- copies of **Acting On Impulse** game cards (pages 110-111)
- copies of **Acting on Impulse** (page 112), one per student
- pencils
- list-making materials—some combination of a whiteboard, markers, different colored index cards, or sheets of butcher paper hung on the wall, etc.

If your students are using *What (Almost) Nobody Will Tell You about Sex*, you can direct them to **Guess Who's Sexually Active** (page 57).

(Pause as the room becomes silent, with every eye riveted on you.)

I've learned that everyone in this room—100 percent of you—are sexually active. [Now would be a good time to smile.]
    Okay, relax, I don't know anything you hope I don't know. I'm just saying there's no such thing as a sexually inactive teenager, because teenagers deal with bubbling hormones and more or less intense sexual desires. All teenagers everywhere are sexually active in the sense that they're growing and making choices about what to do sexually.

Q: Do you agree with this statement? Why or why not?

Q: How does this compare with what most people seem to mean when they talk about teens being sexually active?

Q: Many surveys indicate that a large percentage of teens are sexually active in the sense of having had sexual intercourse. Given who you know at school and at church, do you think that is the case?

Q: To what extent do people in your world talk seriously about gender relationships, hormonal changes, and desire—as distinct from making jokes or rude talk?

        There's a lot of serious conversation

        Here and there, now and then

        Nobody ever treats sex seriously

Q: Do you think it would make a difference if people addressed sex more seriously?

Q: What are some of the things we can do to influence a healthy, ongoing cultural conversation about sex?

To help students reflect further on their own sexuality, use the material included on **Guess Who's Sexually Active** (page 113 in this book) for large group discussion, small group time, or as a tool for individual, personal reflection.

video-driven discussion starter

ESCAPE ROUTE

VIDE

Glorifying God in all aspects of our lives (yeah, including our sexual desires).

This is the scene where Michael Keaton is confronted with a tempting opportunity to have sex with his alluring neighbor, which is made all the more tempting since he mistakenly believes his wife (played by Teri Garr) is having an affair. The most crucial scene is where Keaton is talking to himself in the mirror, making an alphabetical list of the reasons he should go ahead and sleep with the neighbor.
    Set the scene for the *Mr. Mom* clip by explaining that Michael Keaton believes his wife is having an affair, and when the flirtatious neighbor finds out that Keaton thinks this, she decides to pounce.

Q: If Teri Garr's character *were* having an affair, should that influence Michael Keaton's choice? Talk about that.

YOU'LL NEED

• copy of the movie *Mr. Mom* cued to about 1 hour and 21 minutes after the opening 20th Century Fox logo
• television or video projection unit
• VCR or DVD player
• copies of **Escape Route** (page 114), one per student
• pencils

We're not endorsing everything in this movie, we're just saying *this clip* is useful. If that makes you or your boss uncomfortable, let your conscience be your guide.

DESIRE

Q: When you're faced with sexual temptation, what are the things you tend to tell yourself?
- Which of these are helpful? Which are dangerous?
- If your little sister asked you the one thing she should remember when she gets heated up sexually, what would tell her? Why that?

Read 1 Corinthians 10:13.

Q: What stands out for you in this verse?
- Why do you think that's important?
- What difference do you think that could make in your life with your own desires?

Further questions for students' individual personal reflection can be found on **Escape Route** (page 114 in this book).

story and Bible study
HANG ON TO YOUR HORMONES

Counting the costs and rewards of controlling our desires.

Read the following story about Julia to your students.

> "Every Tuesday and Thursday after swim practice, I went to Max's house to hang out. Max's mom worked long hours, so once his older brother went away to college, Max spent most afternoons at home alone. He did homework, watched television, surfed the Internet, and talked every day to his girlfriend Ginny when she had a break from her after-school job at the video store. Ginny didn't mind that Max and I hung out, because Ginny and I had been friends since the fifth grade.
>
> "Max started telling me about all the problems he and Ginny were having. Ginny worked so much that they never had any time together. When they did have time together, she was always so tired that she never felt like doing anything. Even though they talked on the phone every day, Max was getting tired of having a girlfriend he never saw.
>
> "One Thursday, Max was especially angry. He told me all the details of how Ginny had just called him to tell him that she couldn't go out with him on Friday night because—guess what—she had to work.
>
> "Max told me, 'I just wish Ginny was a little more like you and had some more time for me.'
>
> "I started getting a little uncomfortable with Max's compliments, so I went to the bathroom. When I came out I noticed that Max had turned down all the lights and switched the radio to this easy listening, love song station. Max wanted me to sit next to him on the couch, which was where we normally sat when we watched TV, but for some reason it felt different this time. Maybe because the television wasn't on, but I wasn't sure.
>
> "Max put his hand on my hand. I wanted to move my hand, but to be honest, Max's hand felt pretty good. Max leaned against me, putting his head on my shoulder. The lights were dim, the music was soothing, and I was starting to really like how Max's head felt on my shoulder.
>
> "After a few minutes Max started to touch my ear, and then my cheek. I was torn. I knew I should stop him, but it

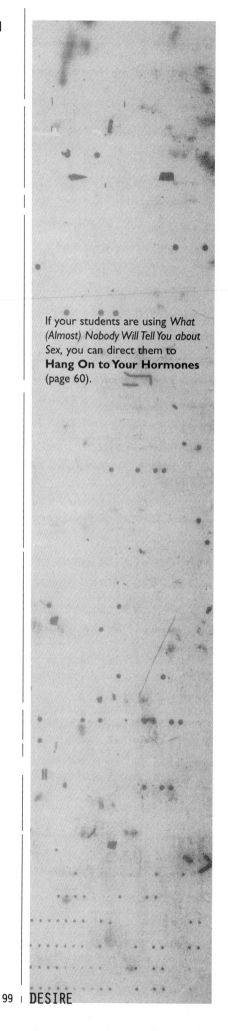

If your students are using *What (Almost) Nobody Will Tell You about Sex,* you can direct them to **Hang On to Your Hormones** (page 60).

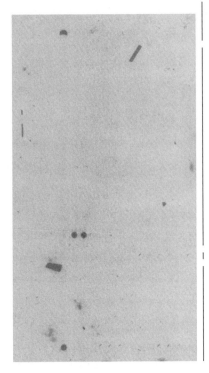

felt so good. Max leaned forward and kissed me on the cheek, and then moved his lips toward mine..."

Q: So what do you think Julia will do? Why?

Someone not too much older than Julia—or you for that matter—was faced with a similar situation.

Read Genesis 39:1-23 with your students. (Consider asking several students to read different sections for the group.) Use the following questions for discussion.

Q: What do you like best about this story? Why?

Joseph must have been pretty good looking because the Bible, which seldom refers to physical appearances, describes him in Genesis 39:6 as "well-built and handsome." It must have run in the family—the only other person in the Old Testament praised for both her figure and face was Joseph's mom, Rachel, who was described in Genesis 29:17 as "lovely in form and beautiful."

Q: Put yourself in Joseph's place. You're a talented, good-looking slave kid who would no doubt like to hang onto your job—not to mention your head. What do you

A note about sexual fetishes

Here and there you'll meet someone with a sexualized obsession toward a nonsexual object or behavior.

I have a friend who is aroused by the sound of spiked heel shoes on a hard floor. As a boy the fantasy of a woman stepping on his hand became attached to his sexual arousal. He doesn't know why.

Another friend is aroused by women smoking cigarettes. He doesn't think he's alone in this, because he found whole Web sites devoted to images of people smoking. He believes his own fascination grew from his parents' preoccupation with the evils of smoking when he was young. The rule in his house—this was in the 1950s—was they had to turn off the sound when a cigarette commercial came on television. He thinks he got the impression that anything that bad might actually be good. (Perhaps this was a trust issue with his parents?)

Another man I know loves women's undergarments. He thinks his appetite for silky things refers back to emotional turmoil from watching his father abuse his mother. His wife told me his lingerie is nicer than hers. It probably goes without saying that puts a strain on their marriage.

A few people are turned on by causing or receiving or observing pain.

All these, and quite a few more, are called fetishes—a term that refers to attaching unwarranted devotion to an object or behavior. There's nothing obviously sexual about these things, yet a few people find them arousing. There may be someone in your group who wrestles with sexual fetishism.

Why do some people have sexual fetishes? I don't know.

My best guess is that fetishism is what Gerald May, author of *Addiction and Grace* (Harper Collins) calls *attraction addiction*. Attraction addictions are marked by all of the following:

- Tolerance—I need more and more to get the same results over time.
- Withdrawal symptoms—I feel bad if I don't get what I long for.
- Self-deception—I lie to myself with excuses, denials, and other mind games.
- Loss of willpower—I don't know how to control my longing.
- Distortion of attention—My longing interrupts love for God, others, and me.

If someone you know struggles with a sexual fetish, you can bet that person feels isolated by the obsession. He is probably emotionally, and perhaps physically, exhausted from the energy expended fighting or hiding what he's up to. And he's afraid—though sometimes he longs to talk with someone about his confusion and pain, even if means being caught. And there's probably another addiction that's more obvious—an addiction to food or making money or spending it or any of a zillion personalized obsessions or think you would think and feel if your owner's wife came on to you?

Q: Are you surprised by Joseph's choices?

Q: Put yourself in Mrs. Potiphar's place. How do you think you would feel if the good-looking slave kid turned down your generous offer of sex?

Q: Put yourself in Mr. Potiphar's place. How do you think you would feel if you came home to find your wife in hysterics, holding the clothes of the good-looking slave kid, claiming he tried to rape her?

In prison Joseph eventually meets people who connect him with the pharaoh. Seeing how talented Joseph is—and it doesn't hurt that God gives Joseph insight into his plans for Egypt—the pharaoh places him in charge of the government where Joseph prepares the whole nation to survive a drought that devastates the rest of the world. I wonder what would have happened if Joseph hadn't refused to have sex with Potiphar's wife.

Q: Do you see any similarities between the story of Joseph and the story about Julia?

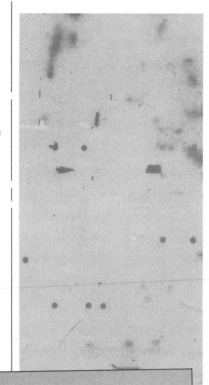

compulsions that obscure the fetish. Which is to say the fetish may not be nearly the most destructive obsession that person deals with, but it may produce the most shame because it's the most unusual.

Because of the characteristics of addiction—tolerance, withdrawal symptoms, self-deception, loss of willpower, distortion of attention—fetishes sometimes lead to increasingly risky, even dangerous, behavior. That's why it's important to try to help people struggling with sexual fetishes.

Which is a challenge in youth groups. Most kids never mention fetishes in youth groups because lots of youth workers make jokes about such things—and who wants to be the butt of jokes? So if you want to serve someone struggling with a sexual fetish, start by not making fun of temptations you don't understand.

To go further, let your group know you're aware that some people struggle with issues they've never heard anybody else talk about. Tell them you're willing to talk in private with anyone who would like to ask questions about temptation or struggle.

Then be prepared for the possibility no one will say anything—or someone may tell you they're the victim of sexual assault; or somebody might talk with you about a "friend;" or who knows what else? The important thing is that you express your openness to any conversation.

Having said that, it's important to acknowledge that if someone does talk with you about a sexual fetish, you probably won't really know what to do. If that's true, do this:

- **Listen compassionately. Ask thoughtful questions. Keep in mind the five marks of addiction above to explore the strength of the fetish. Take your time.**

- **Be honest about the limits of your knowledge and skill.**

- **Reassure him of your commitment to confidentiality and ask if you may put him in touch with someone who has more experience in this area than you. Offer to go with him. See page 13 for some thoughts on referrals.**

- **If the student is a different gender than you are, that's another great reason to ask if you may put him or her in touch with another supportive and caring adult.**

- **If you don't already know who that other helper is, find him in a timely manner and follow through with what you promised. If it takes more time than you thought, let your student know what's going on so he's not left to wonder. Be aware that he'll probably feel pretty vulnerable during this time because the cat is out of the bag.**

- **Follow through. Stay in touch. Don't act as if the conversation never happened. Ask thoughtful questions. Keep confidentiality. Pray for him. And guard your own heart.**

Q: Put yourself in the shoes of the person telling the story that we read before. What are the possible consequences—good and bad—if Julia declines to give in to Max's advances? Be as specific as you can.

Q: What are some possible consequences—good and bad—if Julia gives Max what he wants? Be specific.

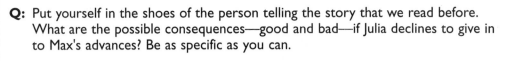

talk and Bible study

SWEET DREAMS ARE MADE OF THIS

Straight talk about lust and what Jesus would say about it.

Alicia, Fox, and Juanita live on the same block and go to the same school. When they were younger, they used to ride bikes together in the neighborhood, but now they've drifted apart. They're into different things at school and have totally different friends now, so they barely say *hi* anymore when they bump into each other between classes or at lunch.

But if you could look into their rooms after school, you'd see they still have a lot in common.

Alicia sits in her bedroom, watching soaps on the TV she talked her parents into buying for her birthday. The people on the screen are undressing each other, though Alicia doesn't actually see them naked, and in the next shot they're under the covers and there's no doubt what they're doing. Alicia's eyes, ears, and emotions are riveted to the screen.

Fox grabs chips and a Mountain Dew, ducks a homework question from his mom, and heads up to his room. He pulls a sports magazine from the lining of his gym bag, but this issue has less to do with baseball and more to do with swimwear—if you catch my drift. He locks the door, flops down on the bed, and opens the magazine.

Juanita sits on her bed, listening to the radio. She can't stop thinking about her conversation with Brad. He is impossibly cute and seemed really interested in what she was doing after school. She wonders what it would be like to go out with him. She closes her eyes and imagines him coming over. She sees herself opening the door and it's Brad, in an oversized sweater and jeans. "Hey," he says, lifting his chin the tiniest bit as he speaks. And a faint smile dances around his eyes.

Q: Do you think Alicia is lusting? Explain your answer.
  • Do you think Fox is lusting? Why?
  • What about Juanita—do you think she's lusting? Why?

Q: Do you believe there's a difference between lusting and merely daydreaming? If so, what is it?

Now read Matthew 5:27-30 aloud—

Q: What do you think Jesus is getting at here?
  • What would you say is his definition of adultery?

A thought about Matthew 5:27-30.
  In verse 27 Jesus quotes Exodus 20:14, but his real goal is to show the true meaning of the commandment against adultery. As he often did, Jesus focuses here on people's hearts, not just their actions. He defines lust as imagining a forbidden sexual relationship. It's doubtful Jesus literally wants people to gouge out eyes or cut off hands if they cause them to sin. We'd all be shy some body

parts in that case. He wants to show that lust is such a radical sin that it requires a radical response. The people who first heard his words would have a shared cultural belief that the right eye and right hand were more valuable than the left, making the consequences of lust even more extreme.

Q: What do you think about this? Why?

Q: Let's ask the questions again. Do you think Alicia was lusting? Why?
- Do you think Fox was lusting? Why?
- Do you think Juanita was lusting?
- When does daydreaming turn to lust?

Q: Do you have any experience with daydreams turning to lust? If so, how do you think it happened?

Q: Do you identify with any of the three characters? Why?

Consider how the following passages relate to that character. Now, read Romans 6:11-13 aloud.

Q: The verb tense of "do not let sin reign" in Romans 6:12 is the present tense, implying that it's a daily, ongoing decision to offer the parts of your body to God instead of to sin. Paul offers no middle ground between offering ourselves to God and offering ourselves to sin. What would "do not let sin reign" mean for the character most like you?

Q: How would your character offer the parts of his or her body to righteousness?

Now read 1 Thessalonians 4:3-5.

Q: Paul describes a difference between people who know God and those who don't. Why does God care about how your character responds to his sexual desires?

Q: If your character wanted to learn from someone else what it means to control his own body, what examples might he or she turn to?

Finally, read Colossians 3:5 out loud.

Q: Any time there's a *therefore* in Scripture, we have to look to previous verses. So we really need to read Colossians 3:1-4 also. Many of the verbs in this passage describe what believers already are—they have died, they have been raised with Christ, their lives are now hidden in Christ. But another verb is used twice to describe what believers should then be able to do, namely set their hearts on things above. Okay, forget about your character and answer for yourself, if you haven't already begun to do so: What do you think it means for you to have died with Christ?
- How do you think setting your heart on things above might affect your sexual imagination?

Q: If you could live in the reality of Colossians 3:1-5, what, if anything, would change in your life?

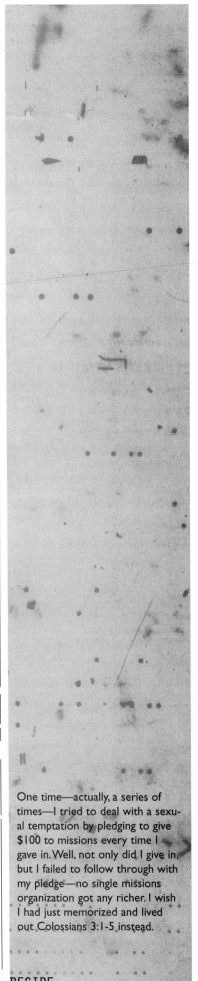

One time—actually, a series of times—I tried to deal with a sexual temptation by pledging to give $100 to missions every time I gave in. Well, not only did I give in, but I failed to follow through with my pledge—no single missions organization got any richer. I wish I had just memorized and lived out Colossians 3:1-5 instead.

If your students are using *What (Almost) Nobody Will Tell You about Sex*, you can direct them to **Is Masturbation Sex?** (page 64).

IS MASTURBATION SEX?

Some of the issues surrounding masturbation.

Okay, so you've heard the word *masturbation*, and maybe even joked about it with others in the school locker room. But do you really know what it is? And have you come to terms with what God might say about it? And how God's opinion relates to your own behaviors?

Let's take one question at a time.

First, what is masturbation? That's probably the easiest one of all. It's touching your own genitals to stimulate yourself and have an orgasm.

Next, what does God say about it? Well, the word *masturbation* never appears in the Bible. Some Christians believe masturbation is always wrong for a few reasons. First, it usually involves visualizing someone of the opposite gender you're not married to, which they would oppose. Second, it is a form of sexual stimulation, and they believe sexual stimulation should be saved for marriage. Other Christians believe it's perfectly all right and normal because teens as well as adults can use it as a way to release sexual pressures. Still others fall somewhere in the middle and say that it may be okay at times, but it can easily become addictive and controlling, so do it only rarely.

One of the issues is that lots of people find that once they start masturbating, they can't stop. Ron had that problem. He had started masturbating in ninth grade, both because of his own curiosity and because it felt good. He did it more often in tenth grade, and pretty much every night in eleventh grade. Now that he's a senior, he's realizing it's starting to control him and he wants to stop.

Well, at least part of him wants to stop. Another part of him enjoys it way too much and wants to do it even more.

So Ron is really confused. He's tried everything he has heard of that might help—taking showers, exercising, avoiding any pictures of girls that might get him thinking about sex—but still he feels trapped.

Q: What would you say to Ron if he asked you what he should do?

Although the Bible never uses the word *masturbation*, it gives us all sorts of principles that help us know what we should do. Let's start with I Corinthians 10:13: "No temptation has seized you except what is common to man. And God is faithful; he will not let you be tempted beyond what you can bear. But when you are tempted, he will also provide a way out so that you can stand up under it."

Q: How does I Corinthians 10:13 relate to masturbation?

Q: Now let's look at James 1:12-15. How do you think masturbation could become a temptation that results in sin?
- Do you believe that it's possible to masturbate only occasionally, unlike Ron who found it became addictive?

Q: Okay, now let's get more personal. Forget Ron. Given I Corinthians 10:13 and James 1:12-15, how do you believe God would want you to act when it comes to masturbation?
- Do you think it's possible that God believes masturbation is okay? If so, why do you think that? When might it become not okay?
- Do you believe it's possible that God would want us to avoid it at all times? If so, why do you think that?

UNTIL I GET MARRIED

Thinking long-term about the consequences of giving in to our sexual desires.

Ahead of time, ask a married member of your adult volunteer team—maybe even you—to share about their sexual experiences and how they relate to desire before being married, and how that has affected their marriage so far. This can be someone who has regrets or someone who doesn't.

> **Most people who want to get married eventually do. And when they get married, they bring not just themselves but also their past sexual experiences into the marriage. Some of you have already had sexual experiences, either by your own choice or not (as in cases of sexual abuse). Some of you regret what you've experienced already. Others want to experience even more as quickly as possible.**
>
> **Since I can't be with you every time you make a decision in response to your sexual desires, my job is to prepare you ahead of time if possible. So I've asked a friend to tell his story. I'll try to give you a chance to ask questions when he's done.**

Q: What's the most important thing that you heard in that story?
   • Why is that important to you?

Q: What difference could this true story make in the way you live out your sexual desires? Why?

Q: If you had the chance to ask a follow-up question, what would that be?

To help your students respond more personally, distribute copies of **Until I Get Married** (page 115 in this book) and pencils and give your students time to reflect and journal about their feelings. Depending on how much time you have, and how vulnerable your students tend to be, you may also want to divide them into pairs to share a few things they've written.

YOU'LL NEED
• copies of **Until I Get Married** (page 115), one per student
• pencils
• married adult volunteer

If your students are using *What (Almost) Nobody Will Tell You about Sex*, you can direct them to **The Lust Factor** (page 63).

CHOICES, CHOICES EVERYWHERE

Read 2 Samuel 11:1-17, then reflect on these questions.

Q: What sexual desires are you experiencing right now? How welcome are they in your life?
- ☐ Entirely welcome because...
- ☐ I could do without them because...
- ☐ I hate them with all my heart because...

Q: What are your options when those desires come on strong?
- • Do you believe your options are limited in any way?
- • What are the consequences—positive and negative—of your different options?

Q: What did you choose the last time you faced those desires? Why?
- • What do you want to choose the next time you face those desires? Why?

Q: With whom can you share this?
- • If you have someone in mind, what do you think you have to gain and lose by sharing with that person?
- • What do you think you have to gain and lose by not sharing with that person?
- • What do you want to do about that?
- • If you don't have anyone in mind, what do you want to do about that?

Choose two guys and two girls to do this skit together. Their lines don't have to be memorized perfectly as long as they can generally follow the script, especially the ending.

Characters
Jessica
Jessica's inner voice
Mario
Mario's inner voice

Setting

A girl and a guy are sitting next to each other in a car. Jessica's inner voice sits in the backseat behind her and leans forward to talk, and Mario's inner voice does the same behind Mario. When Mario and Jessica's inner voices talk, Mario and Jessica should sit as they would if neither of them were talking. Mario drives.

JESSICA: Mario, thanks for taking me to the party. I had a good time.

MARIO: Yeah, me too, especially when Dena tripped over that table. That was hilarious.

MARIO'S INNER VOICE: But my favorite part was when me and Jessica walked in and all my friends were checkin' her out in that little dress. I was just struttin' around. That was cool.

JESSICA: Yeah, I was cracking up when Dena fell.

JESSICA'S INNER VOICE: But I was really checking out Jamie. She always has a date, but tonight she was flying solo, and I was with Mario. She was a sad sight. And I looked fine—if I do say so myself!

MARIO: *(stopping the car)* Well, here we are. So, you wanna talk for awhile or something?

MARIO'S INNER VOICE: I am so good! The car is far enough from her house that her parents can't see but close enough to say we got home on time.

JESSICA'S INNER VOICE: Cool. We're far enough away from the house so Daddy Dearest won't see us. And Mario wants to talk—or something...

MARIO: So, what's up tomorrow?

JESSICA: Well, I'm definitely sleeping in—then my brother has a soccer game. I'm not sure what I'm doing tomorrow night.

MARIO'S INNER VOICE: Was that a hint about tomorrow night? What's she trying to do—own me?

JESSICA: How about you?

MARIO'S INNER VOICE: Careful—I have to sound busy.

MARIO: I've got some family thing tomorrow. I think it's my aunt's birthday or whatever.

MARIO'S INNER VOICE: Perfect. Family-oriented, yet vague.

JESSICA: Yeah, well, we can talk on the phone Sunday. Or maybe in a chat room.

MARIO: *(sliding closer to Jessica)* Yeah, whatever's cool.

(continued)

JESSICA'S INNER VOICE: Pucker up, Buttercup. Don't let him move too fast—but don't look like a prude either!

Mario yawns and stretches and pulls Jessica a little closer.

MARIO'S INNER VOICE: So far, so good. Now stretch, and put your arm around her. Good. Now pull her a little closer. Easy does it. The guys are gonna love this. Except Greg. Greg is gonna be steamed. Sweet!

JESSICA'S INNER VOICE: How's my hair? Oh, my gosh! How's my breath? Gotta be calm and lean in a little. Available, but not too eager.

MARIO: Hey, Jess?

MARIO'S INNER VOICE: This is it. Be cool.

They look in each other's eyes.

MARIO: I was just thinking...

JESSICA'S INNER VOICE: This is it. Be cool.

MARIO: *(leaning closer)* I really like you and all...

MARIO'S INNER VOICE: She looks so hot tonight.

JESSICA'S INNER VOICE: If I kiss him, Winter Formal is in the bag.

MARIO'S INNER VOICE: If I kiss her, she'll expect an invitation to Winter Formal.

JESSICA'S INNER VOICE: If I kiss him, it'll take the relationship to the next level.

MARIO'S INNER VOICE: This is the launching pad. But what if we get going too fast? Am I ready for that?

JESSICA'S INNER VOICE: But I have something to lose here too. Am I ready for that?

Lights out.

BEHIND THE SCENES REFLECTION

Reflect on these questions.

Q: Think about your last sexual experience, however you define that. What do you think was causing you to have that sexual experience?

Q: Try looking a little deeper and harder inside yourself. Often insecurity is behind our sexual experiences. How might that be true, or untrue, for you?

Q: Often fears are what create our insecurities. How might your fears be contributing to your insecurities, which in turn contribute to your sexual desires?

Q: What do you think God might say to you about your fears, insecurities, or desires?
- What makes you think he would say that?

Q: What would you like to do differently, if anything, when you recognize the fears, insecurity, and anxieties that fuel your sexual desires?
- Who could you talk with about what you'd like to do differently? When would be a good time to talk with that person about it?

ACTING ON IMPULSE GAME

Cut these cards apart and use them to play Acting on Impulse (p. 97).

SLEEP 2

CONTACT LENSES 4

POPULARITY 6

TO GET KISSED 1

MONEY 1

TO SCORE A SOCCER GOAL 4

STRAIGHT A's 6

A COMPUTER 2

A CD 3

A DATE 5

A SODA 2

A LETTERMAN JACKET 5

(continue

TO GET MY BRACES OFF 5

TO GO TO A PARTY 2

MOVIES 3

FRIENDS 4

TO GO TO COLLEGE 6

TO WEAR MAKEUP 2

MY DRIVER'S LICENSE 3

MY STEREO 2

THE INTERNET 3

PIZZA 2

MY SKATEBOARD 3

MY MAGAZINES 2

ACTING ON IMPULSE

Reflect on these questions.

Q: What kind of sexual desires are you experiencing these days?
- What other impulses, fears, or other urges might be behind these sexual desires?

Q: Who can you talk to about these other desires or fears?

Q: If you were to read the Bible, what kinds of things do you think it might say to you about these desires, fears, or other urges?

 Write a letter to God about where you could use some help and where you're grateful for the help you've already received.

DEAR GOD,

GUESS WHO'S SEXUALLY ACTIVE

Reflect on these questions.

Q: When do you remember first having sexual thoughts and desires?
  • How did that make you feel?

Q: What do you usually think of when you picture a "sexually active" teenager?
  • Do you fit this category?

Q: Are there other ways that you are sexually active?
  • How do you typically respond to your sexual desires?
  • How do you feel about your typical response?

Q: Are there any ways in which you feel sexually out of control?

 If so, write a letter to God about it. If not, write a letter to God about that.

DEAR GOD,

ESCAPE ROUTE

Write briefly about the following.

• When I'm in the middle of temptation, I tend to...

• One way I could handle temptation better is to think ahead of time about...

• One person I could ask to hold me accountable for my responses to sexual desire is...

• The best time for me to talk to this person on a regular basis is...

• Look at 1 Corinthians 10:13. How does this verse affect your thoughts and feelings about temptation?

Reflect on these questions by yourself or with your group.

 Write a letter to yourself about how you would like to respond to your sexual desires from now until you get married. If you feel stuck, use the questions below.

DEAR ME,

Q: What are your greatest sexual desires and struggles right now?
   • How do you usually respond to those desires?
   • How do you feel about how you usually respond? Why?

Q: What do you believe God would want you to do about your current sexual behavior? Why?
   • In the future, what do you think could make it hard for you? Why?

Q: When your desires are really strong and you're tempted to give in, what do you think you should do? Why?
   • What do you think God can to do to help you? Where did you get your ideas about that?

Q: What's your biggest prayer for your sexual life?
   • If you wish to marry, what's your biggest prayer for your future spouse?

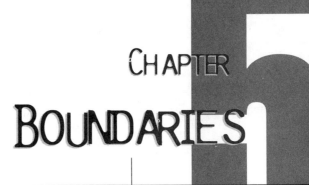

BOUNDARIES

before you teach this lesson...

The Bible doesn't discuss the one question kids most often ask about sex—at least not directly.

The question goes something like this:

I know I'm not supposed to have sex, okay? But how far can I go? Second base? Third base? Not a home run—that would be scoring. But is it okay to get into scoring position?

Well, if sex were a game, that would be an interesting question. The point of games is to get into scoring position in order—at the risk of being obvious—to score. It's bad to finish the inning with runners on base. If sex were a game. But sex is less like a game than a super-intimate conversation. Sex is less like a game than a secret, whispered between husband and wife. Sex is almost sacramental. It's like baptism: the visible sign of an invisible reality.

Fine, but I just wanna fool around a little. How far can I go without getting baptized?

It's a fair question. The trouble is, God doesn't get very detailed about the answer. There's no mention in the Bible of fooling around, nothing about making out. And why is that? Because Bible folk weren't interested in sex? Not likely. Because people got married really young? Umm—maybe. The Bible first spoke into very different cultures than ours, that's for sure.

Fine! Look, I'm just trying to get *a little* without having God all mad at me! So, for crying out loud, will you please just tell me, how far can I go!?

Well, okay. But you may not like the answer because the Bible doesn't really talk about luvsex&dating in any modern sense. What the Bible does talk about—quite a bit, actually—is lust.

So here it is: You may go as far as you wish—as long as you stop before you lust.

Lust is a serious fixation on something that's not ours to have; it's a deep, focused, inappropriate craving. In the Bible, the images associated with lust are heavy breathing, smoldering and bursting into flames. The Bible doesn't talk about hooking up, it talks about longing for experiences that are not rightly ours, and breaking boundaries to get them.

This chapter is about learning to identify and respect sexual boundaries.

The trick is, not everybody lusts the same. Some people can hardly go to an art gallery or ballet without drooling, so forget about watching R-rated films and television. Some people are turned on by the least bit of exposed midriff, so that trip to the beach is going to be a problem. Some people can barely survive a hug, let alone a back rub, so youth group cuddling is just too much to handle. For those who lust easily, just being around other people is a trial; just turning on a computer is a temptation; just going to the pool (or beach or lake) is an ordeal.

Other folks have a much higher lust threshold—who knows why? They take in stride images and touch that drive other people crazy. Which is why Christians are

Boundaries are limits on behavior—what you will and will not accept (boundaries you set with others) and what you will and will not do (boundaries you set with yourself).

called to a high level of sexual sensitivity. It's our duty to look out for each other and do our best to avoid tempting someone who may lust for different reasons than we do.

Now don't go getting all defensive. This doesn't mean girls have to wear clothes that cover from chin to shin. And it doesn't mean boys can't show appropriate affection. It does mean we ought to talk to each other about these things.

Most of us are embarrassed about what makes us lust. We have friends who apparently don't lust at all; they watch videos and read books and dress in ways that drive us over the edge. That's a shameful experience.

So why not give each other a break? Why not ask each other about what triggers lust? This is a dangerous question in one way because it may mean giving up a video from time to time; retiring a favorite outfit because the clerk at Abercrombie wasn't kidding when she said it was hot; hugging side to side instead of belly to belly. And who really wants to give up anything, even for a friend?

But that's the key, isn't it? Friends sacrifice for each other, just because they're friends. And we're not talking about anything that violates your ability to be you. An inconvenience here and there, nothing more.

Turn over the coin. If your group actually decides to ask each other, "What makes you lust?" it's time to speak for yourself. If sexual content on television is a problem for you, please say so. If you fast forward through steamy movie scenes because you know how long those images are embedded in your mind, please share that. And this is okay because you're not alone. We have different thresholds for lust, but sooner or later, we all lust. Anyone who denies that simply hasn't gotten there yet, or they've decided to lie about it. It's just a matter of time.

Whether or not your group has the courage to talk about lust, every individual can and must create boundaries that protect them from lust. If you can't handle seeing people in bathing suits, stay away from places where folks sunbathe. If movies, television, or videos throw you, politely decline to watch them. If the Internet pushes your hot button, move your computer to the kitchen, or at least don't use it behind closed doors. Whatever it takes, okay?

what's in this lesson...

IN OUR OWN WORDS	**WHEN IS IT SEX?** an evaluation opener on what's sexually appropriate outside of marriage
WORD FROM GOD	**YES, MASTER** a Bible study on what happens when Christians behave like pagans
THE LAST WORD	**WHAT DIFFERENCE DOES IT MAKE?** a closing activity that tests your convictions about sexual intercourse
IN OTHER WORDS	See page 124 for additional teaching activities

reflect a moment...

To help your students most effectively, you need to make every effort to process your own sexual experiences, questions, and struggles. Here are some questions to get you thinking:

Q: How did you become aware of the need for sexual boundaries in your life?

Q: Where do you have the greatest difficulty living with your sexual boundaries?

Q: If you are in a friendship with someone who helps you maintain healthy sexual boundaries, reflect on what that person does that is helpful.
- What does that help cost you? Is it worth it?

Q: If you're not in a friendship with someone who helps you maintain healthy sexual boundaries, what do you think you may be missing?
- What do you think it costs you not to have that kind of relationship?
- What do you think it would cost you to find such a person? Do you think it would be worth it?

Q: If you had just one hour to talk with kids about sexual boundaries, what would you try to communicate?
- Why do you think that's so important?
- How would you try to communicate during that hour?

In our own words

video and evaluation opener

WHEN IS IT SEX? —————————————— VIDEO

Identifying the sexual boundaries that seem appropriate outside of marriage.

There are two ways to do this activity—choose whichever one you think will work best for your group and in your situation.

The first option is to create signs before the meeting with the following words or phrases printed on them.

- HUGGING
- HAND-HOLDING
- MASSAGING
- KISSING
- I'LL SHOW YOU MINE, IF YOU'LL SHOW ME YOURS.
- CARESSING
- MUTUAL MASTURBATION
- ORAL SEX
- SEXUAL INTERCOURSE

Post the signs on the wall—or lay them on the floor—in order.
Introduce and show the video clip **"When Is It Sex?"** to your students. Then, without discussing the clip directly, ask the group to move around the meeting area to read the signs. Then, after everyone has a chance to see all the signs, ask them to sit down for a moment so you can explain the next move.

> **What I want you to do is stand near the sign that reflects where you believe you should stop in a dating relationship. The signs are, more or less, in order so pick the first sign that you believe describes an inappropriate sexual act with someone outside of marriage.**

After everyone is more or less settled, ask them to sit down where they are and talk to those sitting with them about why they chose that particular sign. If you feel more comfortable, assign adult leaders to each of the groups to help the discussions along. Then after a few minutes of discussion, get everyone back together again and continue.

If your students are using *What (Almost) Nobody Will Tell You about Sex*, you can direct them to **When Is It Sex?** (page 76).

Option 1

YOU'LL NEED
- VCR or DVD player
- TV or video projection unit
- *Good Sex* video, cued to **"When Is It Sex?"** [26:20]
- signs, made according to directions at left
- tape (optional)
- copies of **When Is It Sex?** (page 131), one per student
- pencils

You can also have your teens do this ranking activity, then show the video and reevaluate their rankings.

Ask for one student volunteer from each of the groups to get up and explain why everyone in that group decided to go to that spot. Follow up with these questions:

Q: Do you agree with the boundaries this group has set? Why or why not?

Q: Is anyone willing to jump ship at this point and join this group?

Go through each of the groups this way, playing the devil's advocate as much as possible to try to get some good discussion going.

The second option is to simply lead the discussion with something like this:

> **I am going to read out a list of activities that are known to occur in relationships. What I want you to do is scream out when you think that what I've just read out is going too far in an unmarried relationship.**

Read out the above list of interactions that happen in a dating relationship, and as students respond according to where they believe inappropriate sexual activity is taking place, ask them why they think that. Promote discussion at all levels of this activity. Play the devil's advocate and stir up debate and thought.

After you have done either of the above activities, ask these questions:

Q: Suppose the person you're going out with has a looser view of when sex begins than you. Whose right or responsibility is it to draw the sexual boundary? Why?

Q: If someone were to ask the majority of people at your school at what point sexual activity is happening, what do you think they would say?

Read 1 Corinthians 5:9-12.

Q: What does this suggest to you about communication with a non-Christian who is sexually active?
  • Is that person held to the same standards as a Christian? Why?

Q: Verse 12 suggests it's none of our business to judge people outside the church. How is that different from not caring what your non-Christian friends do?
  • So if Paul is right here, unless your non-Christian friends are breaking a civil or criminal law, you can't exactly tell them their sexual behavior is "wrong." Can you think of questions you might ask or things you might say to express genuine, loving concern without brining your ongoing conversion about the love of Jesus to a halt?
  • Is there anything that could keep you from doing that for your friends?

Q: Let's write a script together. What would you say if your Christian friend asked you to help him with the words to explain to his non-Christian girlfriend why he won't have sex with her? Not only that, but he thinks some of the things she wants to do are sex—even if she doesn't —and he wishes she wouldn't pressure him.

For even more probing questions about sexual boundaries, use the questions from **When Is It Sex?** (page 131 in this book) for large or small group discussion, or as a tool for personal reflection.

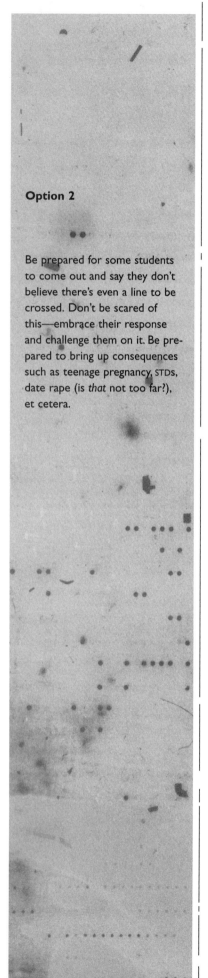

Option 2

Be prepared for some students to come out and say they don't believe there's even a line to be crossed. Don't be scared of this—embrace their response and challenge them on it. Be prepared to bring up consequences such as teenage pregnancy, STDs, date rape (is *that* not too far?), et cetera.

<u>word</u> from<u>God</u>

Bible study
YES, MASTER

What happens when Christians behave like pagans.

Read 1 Corinthians 6:9-11 aloud.

Q: Wow! What do you think Paul is saying?

Q: Some of the really smart folks whose job it is to try and understand the Bible believe that Paul is saying that people who engage in the kinds of sin and sexual acts he describes will not enter heaven. Others believe they can still enter heaven but will not be able to fully experience a relationship with God here on earth. Given what you know about what it takes to enter heaven, what is your opinion?

Q: When Paul says to the Corinthians, "and that is what some of you were" (11), does that have any relevance to this discussion?

In verse 11, Paul talks about three things God does to us and for us when we have a relationship with him. First, he washes us, or spiritually cleanses us. Second, he sanctifies us and sets us apart as his children. Third, he justifies us when he declares us as righteous because of Christ. All of this is made possible because of the work of Christ and the power of the Holy Spirit.

Given all that God has done for us, Paul goes on in the next few verses to talk about how we are to respond.

Read 1 Corinthians 6:12.

Back in the day when this was written, a popular saying in Corinth was, "Everything is permissible for me." These people had taken Paul's message of grace—that it does not matter what we do, God loves us anyway—and turned it into an excuse to do whatever they wanted.

Paul gets in their face about this and says, "Sure, God might not stop loving you, but that does not mean that everything benefits you."

Q: Can anyone think of something that won't cause God to stop loving you but still is not beneficial in your life?

Q: What does it mean to be mastered by something?
  • Can you give an example of something that could master someone?
  • What about an example of something that has mastered you?

Q: Do you think it's true that sexual acts done outside of God's design tend to master people more than anything else? Is this equally true for males and females or more true for one gender?

Read verses 13-14.

Q: Sexual immorality is something we read a lot about in the Bible and hear a lot about in church. What is it?
  • Why are our bodies not made for it?
  • Do you think it's possible to control it?

If your students are using *What (Almost) Nobody Will Tell You about Sex,* you can direct them to **Yes, Master** (page 73).

The culture of Corinth was divided by two major schools of thought regarding the human body. One side believed the human body was so worthless it ought to be thrashed and starved into submission—not a widely popular point of view. The other side believed the body was of little importance compared to the spirit, so they compartmentalized people into body and spirit—separate parts that didn't have much to do with each other. They figured there was no reason to deny their bodies anything they craved since their bodies were destined to go away anyhow, and their real selves were located in their spirits.

121 | **BOUNDARIES**

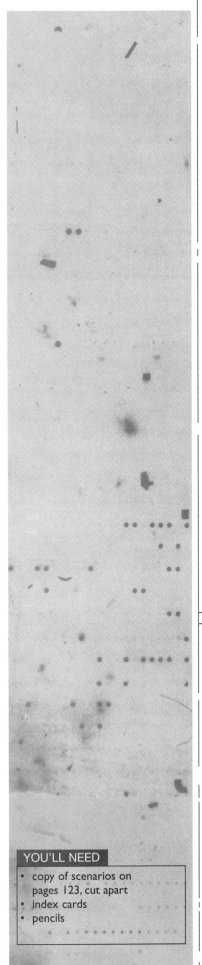

Q: What do you think Paul means when he says our bodies are made for the Lord?

When Paul writes about food and the stomach, he is most likely quoting some Corinthians again (hence the quotation marks in the passage). He seems to agree that things like food and our stomachs are only temporary, but that does not mean anything we do with our bodies is okay. The human body is intended for the Lord and his work.

Read verses 15-20.

Q: The whole concept of our bodies—genitalia and all—belonging to God was a freaky concept for the Corinthians. What does this concept mean to you?

Q: How does seeing our body as belonging to God help us flee from doing the wrong things sexually in our relationships?

Q: What are some things we can do to continually remind ourselves that our bodies belong to God and not us?

Verse 20 is one of the key points in this whole chapter. Paul uses the language of slavery. We were bought like slaves by the death and resurrection of Jesus. Our bodies belong to him, and as a result, we have an obligation to honor him with our bodies.

Q: What do you think it would cost a person if he really, truly honored God with his body?

Q: What do you think that person might get back in return?
  • Do you think it's worth it?

Q: After looking at 1 Corinthians 6:9-20, do you have a clearer answer to the question, How far is too far? If so, what is it?
  • How about a clearer answer to the question, Why would God establish a line he doesn't want us to cross in the first place?

the last word

┌─ closing activity ──────
│ WHAT DIFFERENCE DOES IT MAKE?
└─────────────────────────

A test of convictions about sexual intercourse. Don't worry. No one will be graded.

Give a scenario from pages 122-123 to five leaders and mature students. Get them to read their questions to the whole group. Encourage them to enthusiastically enter into the role of the people they are playing. After each person reads his question out loud, ask the group to give that person solid biblical advice.

After we come to the realization that God does not want anything to become our master and that our bodies belong to him, we have a lot of decisions to make about how we conduct our selves as sexual beings. A few people are going to give us some quick scenarios that raise the question of sexual boundaries. What would you tell each of them?

- I've done everything else. At this point it's just a technicality. What difference does it make?

- I already did it with people I dated before I was a Christian. What difference does it make?

- We've been doing it almost as long as we've been dating. It's too late to turn back. What difference does it make?

- My mother does it with her boyfriend. And I know she expects me to do it, too, because she left a package of condoms on my bed. That's what she thinks of me. So what difference does it make?

- I'm afraid Jesus will come back before I have sex, and I'll miss it. Besides, I know God will forgive me—I mean he has to, he's God. So really, what difference does it make?

Sometimes special circumstances make it seem like it's more okay to cross boundaries that otherwise would be taboo. How would you respond to the following quick scenarios?

- He's going to war and may not come home alive. May I?
- He has cancer—we don't know if they caught it in time. May I?
- We're going to be married in less than a year. May I?
- We're going to be married in less than a week. May I?

Sometimes it's just so hard to say no. We hear so many messages from so many sources that sexual immorality is not only normal, it's expected. Anyone who's decided to follow Jesus has a huge responsibility to stand up and say, "No, my body belongs to God. I am not going to allow sex, or anything else for that matter, to become my master."

Q: What are some of the most convincing arguments that you should not engage in sexual activity?

Q: Is fear a good or a bad motivation for not engaging in sexual activity? Does it work for you?

Q: What are some things that we can do to fight the raging hormones that are yelling at us to become sexually active?

Q: How can we become more accountable to other people for the way we conduct ourselves as sexual beings? Is there someone we can go to when we have issues regarding how far is too far?

At this point, distribute index cards to students and ask them to write down three things:

- How far they choose to go sexually before they get married.
- The reasons they've chosen that point.
- Someone they can talk to about their decision who can hold them accountable—hopefully not just for the next week or two, but all the way until they hear "Here Comes the Bride" at their own wedding.

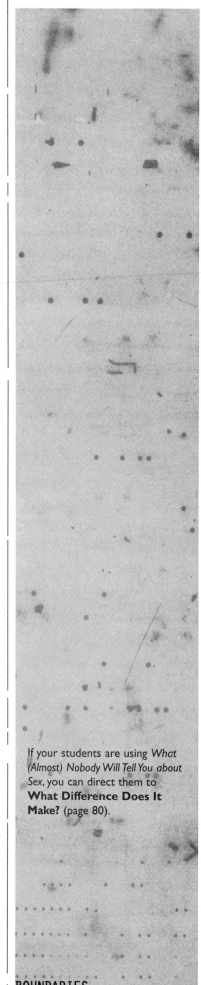

If your students are using *What (Almost) Nobody Will Tell You about Sex*, you can direct them to **What Difference Does It Make?** (page 80).

In other ~~words~~

list-making activity

WHAT IS SEXY?

YOU'LL NEED

- list-making materials—some combination of a whiteboard, markers, different colored index cards, or sheets of butcher paper hung on the wall
- copies of **What Is Sexy?** (page 132), one per student
- pencils

Don't do this exercise if you can't do it in good conscience. It's intended for mature older teens to explore their convictions and the reasons behind those convictions.

If your students are using *What (Almost) Nobody Will Tell You about Sex*, you can direct them to **The Power of Sex** (page 71).

"I'm embarrassed for some of the 'veterans' of music. They had their original [macho] image, and they're still hanging on to it. The sex thing, they're still working it. This-dude-looks-like-your-grandpa kind of thing—it's so silly, it kinda makes you sick. These guys are still using that ancient version of what's sexy, the bikinis and tongues. It's over. I relate to the people that are coming up now, and that's not there, that's long gone.

—*Eddie Vedder, singer and songwriter* (Rolling Stone, October 28, 1993)"

Helping mature students understand the desires of each gender and reflect how that affects the way we treat our brothers and sisters.

Do this opening brainstorming activity by separating the girls from the guys and having two simultaneous discussions and then coming back together to share your results. Or do it together and ask the boys to listen silently while the girls make their list, then ask the girls to listen silently while the boys make their list.

- **Girls, list all the things you think are sexy in boys.**
- **Boys, list all the things you think are sexy in girls.**

Q: Is there anything that surprises you about the other gender's list?

Q: Is there anything that makes you uncomfortable about the other gender's list?

Q: Do you think it's okay to be intentionally sexy if you have no intention of having sex? Discuss that.

Q: What are the potential benefits and risks of recognizing what is sexy?
- Suppose someone is tempted to mishandle the information we've shared about what is sexy. How might they mishandle it? How can we be accountable to each other for handling this conversation responsibly?

For more in-depth personal reflection about what is and isn't sexy, use the questions included in **What Is Sexy?** (page 132 in this book) as guidance for more large or small group discussion, or as a tool for individual, personal reflection.

Bible study

THE POWER OF SEX

Sex is explosive. There. We said it.

Read Genesis 26:1-14.

Q: What do you think of Isaac's strategy to save his own life?
- How do you imagine Rebekah felt about it?
- Would you have gone along if you'd been in Rebekah's sandals?

Look at Genesis 12:10-20 and 20:1-18.

Q: Does any of this sound familiar? Does the phrase *Like father, like son* mean anything to you? Can't you just imagine Isaac sitting around the fire as a boy hearing his dad, Abraham, tell this story?

Look again at Genesis 26:2-5.

Q: What do you think tipped off the king that Isaac and Rebekah weren't brother and sister?

The Hebrew word translated as *caressing* in the NIV, means *playing*. The King James Version of the Bible uses the word *sporting*. It's a word that suggests intimate giggling. Whatever they were giggling

**about when the king looked out his window was something he knew
a healthy guy doesn't do with his sister.**

Q: Do you think Isaac really loved Rebekah? What makes you think that?
- How do you explain Isaac's choice to expose Rebekah to abuse?

Q: Why do you think sex has enough power that men would kill in order to be with
a woman they had no right to be with?

Q: Have you seen anyone hurt because of sex? What happened? How did it turn out?

Q: What things can we do to make sure people we are involved with are not hurt
by the sexual choices we make?

---

another Bible study

WHAT IVORY SOAP HAS TO DO WITH SEX

*A laundry list of inappropriate sex acts and consequences. You'd think most of this would go
without saying, but maybe not.*

Read Leviticus 20:7-24 with your students, then use the following questions for discussion.

Q: Does anything here surprise you?

Q: What do you think the word *consecrate* means?

**In verse 7, consecration is an action by which a person exercises his
will to do God's will. Consecration is also an action to avoid conta-
mination.**

Q: What do you think the word *holy* means?

**In verse 7, holiness is purity. To be holy is to be all one thing, unadul-
terated by anything else. As they used to say, "Ivory soap is 99 and
44/100ths percent pure," which is to say, not quite holy.**

Q: In verse 7, why do you think God calls for consecration and holiness?
- In verse 8, what part does God claim to play in our holiness?
- If this is the case, what part do you think we play in our own holiness?
- From what you've observed, how do you think that's working out in the lives of
  modern people who say they are followers of God? Why do you think that is?

Q: This is a long list of no-nos. What reasons does God give for prohibiting these
behaviors?

Look again at verses 22-24.

Q: Is there anything about God's reasoning here that seems confusing to you?
- God seems to be making an if-then statement. If you do *this*, then *that* will
  happen. Do you believe God's favor is conditional on what we do?

Q: Do you suppose if something isn't on the list in Leviticus 20, that means it's okay?
- What things do you think we could add to this list today?

Q: How do you account for the harshness of the penalty for these acts? I mean, *kill
them* is not exactly the same as *get them in a 12-step group*.

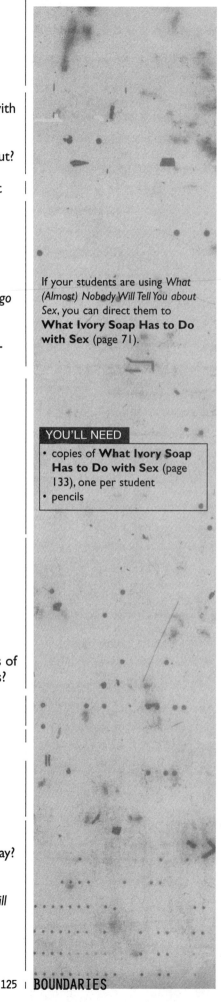

If your students are using *What
(Almost) Nobody Will Tell You about
Sex*, you can direct them to
**What Ivory Soap Has to Do
with Sex** (page 71).

YOU'LL NEED
- copies of **What Ivory Soap
  Has to Do with Sex** (page
  133), one per student
- pencils

Read John 8:1-11 with your students, comparing it to the Leviticus passage. As you discuss John 8, make sure you emphasize that the New Testament does not make the teachings of the Old Testament void. Rather the death and resurrection of Jesus provides a new way for humans to experience God's forgiveness. Since Jesus is the ultimate sacrifice for sin, we no longer have to sacrifice animals, or ourselves, when we sin (and boy, isn't that a great thing?). Instead, we can be purified and justified by repenting for all we've done wrong (see 1 John 1:9). And yet, as John 8 reveals, the forgiveness Jesus offers doesn't give us unlimited freedom to continue in our sinful patterns. As we experience his grace, we should be motivated by our own gratitude to change.

Your Bible probably includes a note that this story isn't in the earliest and best manuscripts. William Barclay comments, in part:

> **Augustine gives us a hint. He says that this story was removed from the text of the gospel because "some were of slight faith," and "to avoid scandal." We cannot tell for certain but it would seem that in the very early days the people who edited the text of the New Testament thought that this was a dangerous story, a justification for a light view of adultery, and therefore omitted it.**
>
> **After all, the Christian church was a little island in a sea of paganism. Its members were so apt to relapse into a way of life where chastity was unknown; and were forever open to pagan infection. But as time went on, the danger grew less, or was less feared, and the story, which had always circulated by word of mouth and which one manuscript retained, came back...we may be sure that this is a real story about Jesus, although one so gracious that for long time men were afraid to tell it.**
>
> **—William Barclay, *The Gospel of John*, Vol. 2. (Westminster Press)**

Q: How does this story compare to Leviticus 20?
- What is similar about the two passages?
- How are the two passages different?

Q: The woman appears to have been caught right in the act. Why do you suppose they brought the woman but not the man to Jesus?

> **One theory holds that they had a special vendetta against the woman; a related theory imagines the man was part of an elaborate trap for her.**
>
> **In verse 5 the accusers quote the Law of Moses—sort of. (Leviticus 20 calls for the man to be executed also.)**
>
> **To further complicate matters, if Jesus said the woman should be executed, he would have allowed the breaking of a Roman law prohibiting execution by local governments. At the same time he would lose his reputation as a friend of sinners (Luke 7:33-35). If he said the woman should simply be let free, it would appear he was counseling them to ignore the Jewish law. What to do?**

Q: What conclusions do you draw from this story?

To help students further process what it means to dedicate themselves to holiness as they experience God's mercy, use the questions from **What Ivory Soap Has to Do with Sex** (page 133 in this book) for additional group or individual reflection.

You'll look at this passage in greater detail in **Do-Overs** (page 166).

" The wages of sin are death, but by the time taxes are taken out, it's just sort of a tired feeling.
—*Paula Poundstone, comedienne* "

Alcohol + sex = ???

Read the following story to your students.

> I've had friends who used alcohol as an excuse to go farther than they said they would. Others were taken where nobody wants to go because they were drunk.
>
> "I had too much to drink," they say. "I'm not sure how it happened."
>
> I've even heard friends say, "I'm not sure what happened. I hope I didn't do anything bad."
>
> One friend was raped by several boys at a party while she was under the influence. She woke up the next morning sore and hung over. When she realized what had gone on the night before, she freaked out and spent several days in a psychiatric hospital. It's been hard for her to come back from that experience.
>
> Another friend was raped when she lost at Quarters, a drinking game that involves flipping coins into shot glasses—the loser of each round drinks the shot. Her friend, who invited the boys to her house after school, managed to fight off the boy who attempted to rape her. But my friend was too far gone to fight the boy who climbed on top of her. The girls were so ashamed and afraid of getting in trouble with their parents that they never told anybody. Well, that's not quite true—my friend told me about this incident while in the hospital after narrowly surviving a suicide. This most serious attempt on her life came after several years of bulimia and sexual craziness. It was another half decade before she started to live a normal life, more or less.
>
> Sometimes I wonder what it is that makes some people prefer to not know—or not seem to know—what they're doing sexually. And what is it about alcohol that can put people in a position where they can't defend themselves?

Q: Does this story sound familiar? How so?

Q: What do you think is going on with males or females who drink so they have more nerve to get into sexual activity?

Q: Have you ever seen that work out well for anyone?

Q: What opinions have you formed about guys who drug girls with alcohol or other substances in order to rape them?

Q: Do you think those boys believe it's rape? Talk about that.

Q: Do you believe it's rape?
  • Yes because...
  • No because...

Read Romans 13:9-14 with your students.

Q: How do you think this passage applies to the "I was drunk" excuse?

Q: How do you think this passage applies to a guy who uses alcohol or another drug to set up a girl?

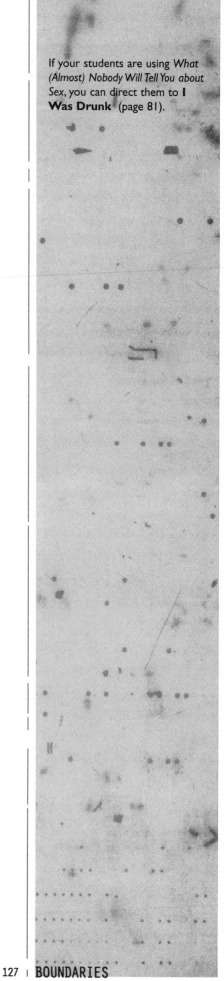

If your students are using *What (Almost) Nobody Will Tell You about Sex*, you can direct them to **I Was Drunk** (page 81).

The implication of verse 14 puts the emphasis on thinking ahead about how to gratify ourselves wrongly.

Q: What percentage of sexual encounters do you think really just happen with no forethought, no planning, and no setup by either party?

0% because...   50% because...   100% because...

case study
BEING "CAREFUL"

The need to be "careful," but in the right way.

Read the following story aloud to your students.

> **A few months after his prom night, my friend Jim told me what it was like for him to have sex the first time: "I guess there wasn't really a moment when I decided, but it was like a process of decisions leading up to it. I'd been going out with this girl for a few weeks. Our physical relationship got way ahead of everything else—we hardly even talked sometimes. I figured sex might just happen, if the night was good enough—and prom night is usually kind of special.**
>
> **"I know I needed to be 'careful' so I bought my first condoms. So that's a big step for me, I guess. And when it finally came down to it, it was kind of clinical, actually—there were so many more factors that went through my head. I needed to find a place and a time. A place where we could get alone and no one would find out. It ended up being some kind of an operation, where I had to take care of a whole bunch of logistical factors instead of just letting that moment I'd planned on take control.**
>
> **"I was really at odds with what I was believing and what I was doing. They were two totally different things."**

Q: What stands out for you about this story?

Q: What do you think he meant at the end by saying what he was believing and what he was doing didn't match up?

Q: What do you think of the argument that says, "If you can't be good, at least be careful"?
   • What do you think people mean when they talk about being careful?

Q: What do you believe God thinks about that?

> **If you think about the word *careful*, it basically means being full of care. It's too bad that when it comes to sex, being careful has been reduced to making sure you use some form of protection during sex. In reality, being careful should mean being full of care for the people involved in your sexual decisions—meaning yourself, the other person—oh, and God.**
>
> **And here's a mind-blowing thought. What if you based your sexual actions on what was the best and most caring thing for your future spouse? How might that affect the sexual boundaries you create for yourself?**

If it feels appropriate, give students some time to reflect on what kind of stories they'd like to be able to tell their future spouse about all of their sexual behavior leading up to their wedding night. For students who have already had sex, remind

If your students are using *What (Almost) Nobody Will Tell You about Sex*, you can direct them to **Being "Careful"** (page 80).

them how inspiring it would be for them to be able to tell their future spouses that although they made some mistakes early on, by God's grace, they had the strength to eventually make better choices.

list-making activity

WHY WAIT?

Evaluating whether or not to postpone sexual involvement until we're married.

> • **List as many reasons you can think of for delaying sexual intercourse until marriage.**
>
> • **List as many reasons you can think of for having sex early and often.**

Q: Which reasons are most convincing to you? What makes them persuasive?

Q: Which reasons are least convincing to you? Why are you unconvinced?

To help students crystallize their personal convictions about sex, use the questions from **Why Wait?** (page 134 in this book) for group or individual reflection.

brainstorming discussion activity

10 WAYS TO SAY NO

How to say no even if a little part of you wants to say yes.

> **List as many ways as you can think of to turn down someone who wants to take you farther sexually than you want to go.**

Q: Do you think it's equally difficult for every person to hit the brakes sexually? Why or why not?
  • Do you think there are some situations that make hitting the brakes more difficult? Why do you think that's so?

Q: Do you think there's a progression of sexual contact that's assumed by most people when they're going out? In other words, is there a set order to how a relationship develops sexually?

If the group believes there's an assumed progression, write it where everyone can see. Then ask—

Q: How soon in a relationship do you think most people would expect each of these sexual experiences?

Q: What makes you think what we're saying here is more or less true?

Q: Where do you think these sexual expectations come from?

Q: Do you think one gender drives these expectations more than the other? Why? How do you feel about that?

To help students continue to process how to respond to sexual pressures and establish healthy boundaries, use the questions from **10 Ways to Say No** (page 135 in this book) as material for large or small group discussions, or as a tool for individual personal reflection.

YOU'LL NEED
• list-making materials—some combination of a whiteboard, markers, different colored index cards, or sheets of butcher paper hung on the wall
• copies of **Why Wait?** (page 134), one per student
• pencils

YOU'LL NEED
• list-making materials—some combination of a whiteboard, markers, different colored index cards, or sheets of butcher paper hung on the wall
• copies of **10 Ways to Say No** (page 135), one per student
• pencils

If your students are using *What (Almost) Nobody Will Tell You about Sex*, you can direct them to **Mother, May I?** (page 78).

WHEN IS IT SEX

Q: When do you believe it's sex? Identify the behavior you think is the threshold of sex between two people.

☐ Hugging   ☐ Hand-holding   ☐ Massaging

☐ Kissing   ☐ I'll show you mine if you'll show me yours

☐ Caressing   ☐ Mutual masturbation   ☐ Oral sex

☐ Sexual intercourse

• How did you reach that conclusion?

Q: Have you had a disagreement about that with anyone you were involved with?
• If so, what happened?
• How did you feel?
• How did you work it out?
• How do you feel toward that person now?

**W
H
E
N**

Q: Do you think there's a way to find out what a person's view of sex is without having a wrestling match?
• How could a conversation about what sex is be helpful to two people in their dating relationship? Can you think of any harmful effects?
• Do you think you can go out with someone who has a different view of sex without somebody getting hurt? Why?

Q: Do you think it might be helpful if you could compare notes with someone on this?
• What do you think you have to lose and gain by doing that?

WHAT IS SEXY?

Reflect on these questions.

Q: Is there anything you find sexy that you would have difficulty telling to your group?
- Why do you think that's difficult to talk about?

Q: Can you recall the first time you found that thing appealing?
- What was going on in your life at the time?
- Can you recall what it is or was about that thing that appealed to you?

Q: What's your current feeling about that thing you find sexy but can't easily talk about?

Q: Do you ever feel isolated because you find that thing sexy?
- If so, try to think of one person you can trust with this secret.

Reflect on these questions by yourself or your group.

Read Leviticus 20:7-24 and John 8:1-11 and then reflect on these questions.

Q: How do you feel about the tension between punishment and mercy for sexual wrongdoing in the Bible?
    • Where do you tend to come down on the scale?
  ☐ Punishment because...   ☐ Tolerance because...   ☐ Mercy because...

punishment —|—|—|—|—|—|—|—|— mercy

• Why do you think you've landed at that point on the scale?
• If you had to land on one side of the scale or the other, where would you want to be?
• When God looks at your life, where do you believe God lands on this scale?
  What makes you think that?

Q: Do you know anyone who's really in need of mercy from God because of sexual wrongdoing?
    • If so, why do you think they need mercy?

Q: Do you know anyone who needs to show mercy for sexual wrongdoing?
    • If so, why do you think they need to show mercy?
    • What do you think it would cost that person to show mercy?
    • What do you think he has to gain by showing mercy?

WHY WAIT?

Reflect on these questions.

Q: Have you decided what you will and won't do sexually in a relationship?
  • How did you develop those beliefs?

Q: Have your current convictions been tested?
  • How did you resolve that challenge?

Q: What do you think, if anything, it would take to change your convictions?

Q: Is there anybody else who knows about some of your decisions about sex?
  • How can you remain accountable to that person for the decisions you've made?

10 WAYS TO SAY NO

Reflect on these questions.

Q: How do you feel about sexual expectations in your relationships?

Q: If anyone has ever put you in an unfair spot, how did it begin?
- What happened next?
- And then?
- What was going on inside you?
- Has it been resolved? Why?
- What is your relationship with that person today?
- How do you feel about that experience now?

Q: If you ever put someone in an unfair spot, how did it begin?
- How did it unfold?
- What was going on inside you?
- Has it been resolved? Why?
- What's your relationship with that person today?
- How do you feel about that experience now?
- Now that you've put someone in an unfair spot, do you think you're more or less likely to do it again? Why or why not?

Q: If you were to view others as brothers or sisters in Christ, would that affect how you treat them sexually? Reflect on that a bit.

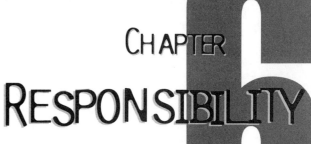

before you teach this lesson...

Like it or not, each of us is responsible for our sexual behavior. *Acting* as if that were true, actually taking responsibility, is what this chapter is about.

It's like the rules of the road. Every state has some version of the Basic Speed Law, which states that motorists may drive only as fast as is reasonable under prevailing conditions. That means drivers must slow down on wet or slippery pavement, regardless of the posted speed limit, and no matter what others do. "Everyone else was driving 65" is interesting but won't clear you if you skid into a car on a slick highway. You still get the moving violation, and if you're lucky, that's all you get.

"Everybody does it" is no excuse for behavior that violates the Basic Speed Law of sexuality. You're not responsible for "everybody."

It's not hard to understand sexual responsibility. Just ask, What are the prevailing conditions of my life? Given these conditions, What is responsible sexual behavior?

Yeah, but you don't understand my situation: I'm not a slut or anything, but... Maybe I'm just hornier than most people.

That's an interesting theory, but if someone gets hurt, you're responsible for your behavior.

But you don't understand—my girlfriend is really hot. I can't control myself.

Sorry, but if you lose control, that just means you're driving too fast for prevailing conditions.

But, seriously, I think about sex all the time. That is my prevailing condition. Why would God give me hormonal urges and then tell me not to fulfill them? That's just mean.

It's not mean; it's a measure of human responsibility. If we were just like the other animals, things would be different. We're not. Humans are all that and a bag of chips. We have the capacity—or should we say, a responsibility—to live above our basic instincts, and doing so enriches our deeper selves.

About now you may be saying, *Fine, I'm responsible. Tell me to whom and for what, and I'll give it a shot.*

Fair enough.

- We're responsible to *God* because God made us and we belong to God before we belong to ourselves or anyone else.
- We're responsible to *each other* because we are brothers and sisters before we are anything else on the earth.
- We're responsible to *ourselves* because even if we don't understand it, we long to become what God made us to become.

The apostle Paul says this.

"It is God's will that you should be holy; that you should avoid sexual immorality; that each of you should learn to control his own body in a way that is holy and honorable, not in passionate lust like the heathen, who do not know God; and that in this matter no one should wrong his brother or take advantage of him. The Lord will punish men for all such sins, as we have already told you and warned you. For God did not call us to be impure, but to live a holy life."
(I Thessalonians 4:3-7)

Responsibility means living with appropriate boundaries and making amends when you cross the line—both of which are learned skills and neither of which is easy.

Paul's definition of sanctification here is avoiding sexual immorality, learning to control our bodies in a way that's holy and honorable, and doing no harm to our sisters and brothers. You may not have to look any further than your own youth group to see out-of-control people taking advantage of their brothers or sisters in Christ. Pity.

Paul spins it another way in a letter to the church at Rome. "Let us behave decently, as in the daytime, not in orgies and drunkenness, not in sexual immorality and debauchery, not in dissension and jealousy. Rather, clothe yourselves with the Lord Jesus Christ, and do not think about how to gratify the desires of the sinful nature" (Romans 13:13-14).

It's a vivid image. People who put on Christ have a fighting chance at thinking about more than just how to gratify their own desires. For people who aren't clothed with Jesus, it's more of an uphill battle.

A lot of kids lose that fight every day. They live in an endless spiral of determination, failure, resolution, failure, recommitment, failure, remorse, failure—all because they think clothing themselves with the Lord Jesus Christ means asking, "What would Jesus do?" and then attempting to behave as decently as they can on their own. Which, it turns out, is not all that decent. It's not that they're worse than other kids, it's just that, to grab a phrase from Jesus, "apart from me, you can do nothing."

If students are going to win the fight, their only hope is to ask Jesus to help them win it. That takes a more thorough conversion than many have yet experienced.

But then they need to ask others to help them also. Along with a deepening intimacy with the God who alone can sanctify and make us holy, acting responsibly takes support and accountability in the community of God's people.

what's in this lesson...

IN OUR OWN WORDS

THIS IS A TEST an evaluation activity about sexually transmitted diseases

WORD FROM GOD

U DA MAN! a Bible study on being sexually responsible before God and others

FIGHTING FIRES a video discussion starter on how Christians must help each other cope with sexual struggles

THE LAST WORD

TALK ABOUT IT a closing application on choosing people to hold us accountable

IN OTHER WORDS

See page 144 for additional teaching activities

reflect a moment...

To help your students most effectively, you need to make every effort to process your own sexual experiences, questions, and struggles. Here are some questions to get you thinking:

Q: What are some of your most rewarding experiences of sexual responsibility?
• Describe the cost of taking responsibility on that occasion.

Q: What are some of your most significant failures to take sexual responsibility?
• How do you think that happened?
• What did you learn about sex? About yourself? About God?

Q: If you had just one hour to talk with kids about sexual responsibility, what would you try to communicate?
- Why do you think that's so important?
- How would you try to communicate during that hour?

In our own words

If your students are using *What (Almost) Nobody Will Tell You about Sex*, you can direct them to **This Is a Test** (page 92).

= evaluation activity

THIS IS A TEST

The extent of sexual diseases, and the ramifications for acting responsibly.

Set up a continuum of 11 stripes of tape on the floor, or 11 chairs, or 11 sheets of paper on the wall. Label from zero to 100 percent, according to the following example—

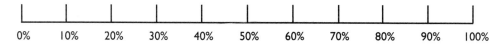

0%   10%   20%   30%   40%   50%   60%   70%   80%   90%   100%

As I ask each question from this fact sheet, stand beside the percentage marker you believe to be closest to the correct answer.

Read the first question on **This Is a Test Fact Sheet** (page 158). After your students move to where they think the answer will be, read the answer. Congratulate the students who got it right by throwing them some candy. Continue through the other questions. Have your students sit back down and ask these questions.

YOU'LL NEED
- marker
- candy
- paper
- masking tape
- 11 chairs
- copy of **This Is a Test fact sheet** (page 158)
- copies of **This Is a Test** (page 159), one per student
- pencils

Q: If a person knew he were infected, what obligations do you believe he would have to anyone he went out with? Why?
- What percentage of infected individuals do you think live up to those obligations? Why do you think that?

Q: Have you ever heard of anybody in your peer group going for a blood test to find out if they might be carriers of an infectious disease? How did they feel? What advice would you want to give?

Q: Given what you have just heard about the extent of sexual diseases, how likely do you think it is that you know someone who has one?
- If you have a suspicion that someone's sexual behavior might lead to a sexual disease, what's your responsibility to that person?
- If that person *does* have a sexual disease, then what is your responsibility to him?

To help students dive even deeper into the reality of sexually transmitted infections and their responsibility, use the questions from **This Is a Test** (page 159 in this book) for additional group discussion or personal reflection.

word from God

= Bible study

U DA MAN!

YOU'LL NEED
- copies of **U Da Man!** (page 151), one per student
- pencils

We're responsible to God and to others for our sexual choices.

Read 2 Samuel 12:1-13.
Before you begin this section of the study, do a quick recap on the story that inspired this little visit from Nathan. See 2 Samuel 11.

If your students are using *What (Almost) Nobody Will Tell You about Sex*, you can direct them to **U Da Man!** (page 87).

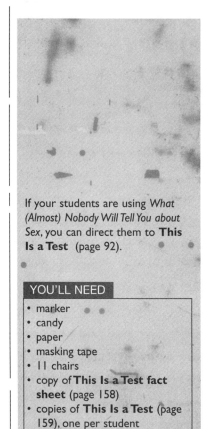

One easy way to define the word *responsibility* is the *ability* or *requirement to respond*. Basically that means that you are expected to act, and it's assumed that you're going to act, in a way that is best for all involved, not just yourself. It's just common sense. If you're a responsible babysitter, you won't leave a two-year-old alone all day. If you're a responsible student, you'll study what your math teacher tells you to study.

Being responsible also relates to our sexuality. Using the story of David, today we're going to look at two levels of responsibility we all share when it comes to our sexuality:
• God
• Others

——— Our responsibility to God

Q: Do you believe it was right that David was set up like this by Nathan?

Q: Try to put yourself in David's shoes for a moment. How would you feel if you were hearing that stuff said right out loud?
• Would you be angry with God that he told Nathan about your personal life?

Q: How would you feel if your youth leader-pastor-minister went toe to toe with you over a sin God told him you committed?

David was a man specifically chosen by God as a special servant. That kind of choosing carries some pretty serious weight. David could not just go around and do whatever he wanted—he had a responsibility to the one who had chosen him and blessed him beyond measure.

Q: In what ways do we have a responsibility to God for our actions in general?

Q: When it comes to sex, what responsibility do we have to God?

Q: David suffered severe punishment for neglecting his responsibility to God. When we do the same thing, what happens to us?

——— Our responsibility to others

Read 2 Samuel 12:1-25.

Q: What I want us to do is go through this passage (verses 1-25) and count all the people who were affected by David's actions. How many were there?

ANSWER: Uncountable

Here is the cast of characters who were affected by David's irresponsibility as I count them in this passage:

• God (verses 8-9)
• Uriah the Hittite (9)
• Bathsheba, wife of Uriah (10)
• All of David's wives (11)
• Son born to Bathsheba and David who dies (14)

Include in this list all the people of Israel who lost faith in their king as a spiritual leader because of this act, and you have an uncountable number of people affected by David.

Q: Can you think of another time when the sexual actions of one person affected a lot of people?

If you think you still need to reinforce the point that the sexual actions of one person can affect a whole bunch of people, share the following illustration.

Back in the 1980s, excess was in (along with tight jeans and the color turquoise, but that's a longer story). In the minds of many, the more you had the better you were. Televangelists built minikingdoms for themselves on the backs of people they begged money from, promising them financial return for money they gave. A lot of people found their hope and eternal security in these men—never a good thing to do.

These kingdoms crashed when reporters and photographers snapped pictures of some of these men leaving hotels with prostitutes and secretaries. Only God can judge the actions of these men, but we can look back and see the damage their sexual irresponsibility caused. To this day many people have a deep mistrust for ministers of the word of God because of the foolishness of these men.

But they were just like David. They thought for the moment and not for the long term. This brought a whole lot of trouble, not just to them, but to all who called themselves Christians.

Q: We've spent some time looking at how the sexual choices we make often have negative consequences for others. Could the opposite also be true—that the choices we make often have positive consequences for others? Can you give an example of this?

Read the following account to your students as an example of the way our decisions affect others.

> A few years ago, a college student told me she was pregnant, and I was the only one who knew. As we talked, it became clear she wanted an abortion, but she didn't want to face that alone. She was no longer in contact with the father of the child. I suppose she felt pretty isolated. Finally, she asked if I would go with her to the clinic.
>
> I said no. I told her my theological reasons and tried to convince her to look for another way. When the conversation ended, I guess neither of us felt like we got what we wanted from the other.
>
> A few days later, her sister came to town and agreed to take her to the clinic for the procedure. I always thought she made the wrong choice, but I've never been certain I made the right one.
>
> Was I as convincing as I could have been about my church's willingness to help her through the pregnancy, maybe help her with an adoption—whatever it might take to stand by her? Would she have made a different decision?
>
> What if I had offered to go with her? What if she had agreed to wait a while before making a final decision? Would that have given her more time to think about it? Would she have made a different decision?
>
> Who knows?
>
> I just know I never felt like I handled that very well. I mean, she had the abortion, right? I don't know. I would wish for another chance on this one, but honestly, I'm not 100 percent sure what I would do.
>
> I feel bad about that, too.

Imagine that right now a young woman we know is sitting in a coffee shop, wondering what to do about being pregnant. Let's say we knew she was coming to us with this problem one week from today.

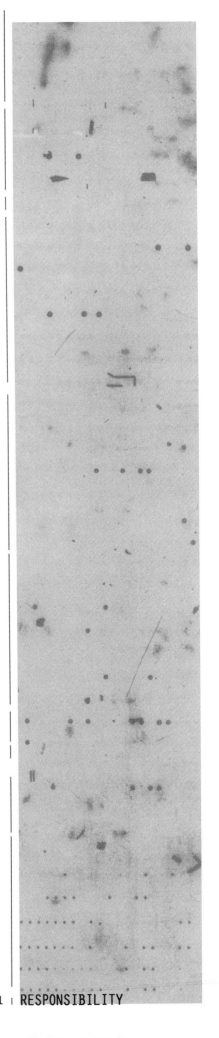

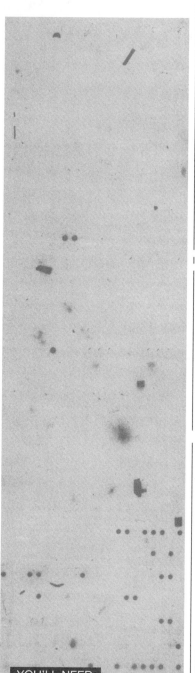

Q: What would you want to be prepared to say to her?
  • Is there anything that would keep us from saying that? Why?

Q: Do you think going to the abortion clinic with her shows responsibility or irresponsibility toward her? How about toward God?

Back to the story of David. We've already seen how he didn't act responsibly toward others, but the flip side of the story is someone who acted very responsibly. The prophet Nathan really stepped up to the plate in this situation and bore the responsibility to confront the king. This must have been a scary thing to do—he could have lost his life; he knew David had already killed to cover up his mistake.

Q: What are some things we can do to step out of our comfort zones and act responsibly when others are making sexual choices that seem to go against what God wants?

Q: Are there any boundaries we would cross by doing this? Is this a bad thing?

One of the often overlooked elements of this story is what Nathan did after he confronted David. In 2 Samuel 12:25, we see that when Bathsheba has another son (Solomon), Nathan the prophet is the one who announces his birth—and that the name Jedidiah will be attached to this son, meaning that this son is loved by the Lord. After Nathan acted responsibly and confronted David about his sin in the whole Bathsheba-Uriah mess, he didn't just split. He stuck around and was part of God's redemption for David. He really understood his responsibility to David.

Q: If you wanted to act as responsibly as Nathan in the story about the college woman who had the abortion, what would you do?
  • What would make it hard to do that?
  • Given those difficulties, what would motivate you to stay in the woman's life?

To help students personalize the story of David and Nathan, use the material from **U Da Man!** (page 151 in this book) as background for large or small group discussion, or as a tool for individual, personal reflection.

┌─video discussion starter──
│ **FIGHTING FIRES** │────────────────────────────────────── ┐ **VIDEO**

The responsibility of a Christian community to help each other with our sexuality.

After you show the **"Fighting Fires"** video clip, lead the following discussion.

Q: Okay, a little hint here. The video is a parable about something deeper. And since this is a book about sex, it might not come as a big surprise to hear it's something related to sex. What do you think a *sexual fire* is?

Q: What kinds of things do you think stop a guy like Andy, or a person like any of us, from acting responsibly and fighting sexual fires that others are going through?

Q: What do you think Andy—the firefighter who doesn't fight fires—has to say to a group like ours?
  • Andy was surrounded by signs of fires. Is that true for us? Do you feel surrounded by sexual fires?

YOU'LL NEED
• list-making materials
• television or video projection unit
• VCR or DVD player
• *Good Sex* video, cued to **"Fighting Fires"** [28:45]
• copies of **Fighting Fires** (page 152), one per student
• pencils

This discussion is going to get more and more confusing if your students lack some sort of shared definition of sexual fires. What *we* mean by "sexual fires" is sexual struggles people are going through.

Do you think we could be ignoring sexual fires in our Christian community? If so, let's make a list of the kinds of fires you see. I'll go first—I see signs of sexual abuse, how about you?

After you have a list of these fires, follow with—

Q: Do you think a person can help others fight sexual fires before she gets her own fire under control? Why or why not?

Q: Andy had the tools and education to fight fires, but he lacked the will. Do you think we have the tools we need to fight the sexual fires around us?
  * If so, what are those tools?
  * If not, what are the tools you think we need to do the job?

Q: At least part of Andy wanted to fight fires. Do we really want to address the sexual fires in our lives and in the lives of the people around us?
  * It's possible that Andy was afraid of fighting fires. Is fear ever a motivation for not wanting to accept responsibility for the sexual fires that rage around us?
  * What might happen if we hop in to fight other people's fires when they don't ask us to? Is this ever a good thing? Why or why not?

Q: Eventually Andy was fired—firefighters have to fight fires, right? How about us— what could happen to this group if we fail to help ourselves and other people whose houses are burning down?

To help students focus more closely and personally on dealing with the sexual fires around them, use the questions from **Fighting Fires** (page 152 in this book) for large or small group discussion, or individual, personal reflection.

the last word

closing application

TALK ABOUT IT

Choosing who we can ask to encourage and hold us accountable as we struggle with sexual responsibility.

> **There's an old saying among recovering addicts—"We are only as sick as our secrets." I believe that's really true as we discuss our responsibility to God and others. We have a responsibility to deal with the things that cause us to live in shame and guilt.**

Q: What do you think makes people hold onto their secrets and keeps them from sharing their struggles so others can help?

Q: Is this what keeps you from sharing struggles?

Read the following quote to your students from Dietrich Bonhoeffer. He believed this is how Christians should think about each other:

> **Even Paul said of himself that he was the foremost of sinners (1 Timothy 1:15)...There can be no genuine knowledge of sin that does not lead to this extremity. If my sinfulness appears to me to be in any way smaller or less detestable in comparison with the sins of others, I am still not recognizing my sinfulness at all. My sin is of necessity the worst, the most grievous, the most reprehensible...My sin is the worst...How**

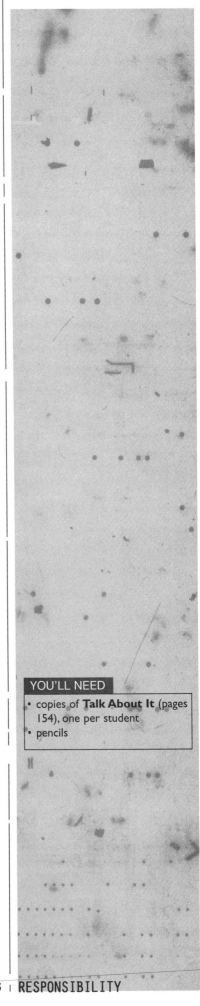

YOU'LL NEED
* copies of **Talk About It** (pages 154), one per student
* pencils

can I possibly serve another person...if I seriously regard his sinfulness as worse than my own?
—Dietrich Bonhoeffer, *Life Together* (Harper and Row)

Q: How big do you believe your sin is in comparison with others?

Q: What responsibility do you believe you have in sharing your sinfulness with God and others?

Q: If you sense someone else is struggling with a sexual issue, what responsibility do you have to them?

Q: What are some things you can do to become more responsible to God when it comes to your sexual questions and struggles?

Q: What are some things you can do to become more responsible toward others when it comes to your sexual questions and struggles?

Q: What are some things you can do to learn personal responsibility and how every action has either positive or negative consequences?

Conclude this exercise by distributing pencils and copies of **Talk About It** (pages 153-154 in this book) to each student. After giving them several minutes to complete the handout, have them huddle in groups with one or two other students to share one thing they've learned from this discussion and one way that will impact their sexuality.

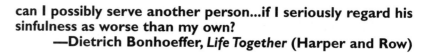

In other words

┌─video opener
│ **TROUBLE** ├──┤**VIDEO**

Signs that a friend might be in relational trouble.

Q: What strikes you about this video clip?
  • Have you seen any of these signs of trouble in a relationship? If so, and without embarrassing anyone, talk about what you've seen or experienced.

Q: Do you think most people don't recognize trouble signs when they see them or do you think most people ignore signs of trouble? Discuss that.
  • How do you think some people miss what seem to their friends like clear signs of trouble?
  • Why do you think some people ignore the warning signs?

Q: There's an old saying that love is blind. There's a somewhat newer saying that love is not blind, love is stupid. Do you agree or disagree?

Q: What responsibility do you think friends have to each other before, during, or after signs of trouble appear in a relationship?

• Before

• During

• After

YOU'LL NEED
• four student volunteers
• a television or video projection unit
• VCR or DVD player
• *Good Sex* video, cued to **"Trouble"** [31:35]

To "listen" another's soul into a condition of disclosure and discovery may be almost the greatest service that any human being ever performs for another.
—Douglas Steere, Gleanings: A Random Harvest (Abingdon, out of print).

LINE UP

The influence of people around us.

Ahead of time, secretly ask eight students to raise their hands when you ask for volunteers to play Line Up. Explain that they should play along and say that Line A is longest.

Ask for 10 volunteers, the eight you have secretly prepared in advance plus two other real volunteers. Send four of your prepared volunteers and one real volunteer out of the room beyond earshot. (You may want to ask an adult to hang out with them so they end up far enough not to hear, but closer than the donut shop down the next block.)

Show the five remaining volunteers the lines you drew and "randomly" call on them to pick which line is longest. Of course there's nothing random about it, because you'll choose your four prepared volunteers first and your real volunteer last.

After the deed is done, show the lines to the group and explain that you prepared four volunteers ahead of time to see how the fifth person would respond.

Now the group is in the know for round two and the next five volunteers. Repeat the process, choosing your four prepared volunteers first and your real volunteer last.

After the game is over, ask the two volunteers who were not prepared in advance—

Q: How did you start to feel as you heard the other four answers?
  • Why did you answer as you did?
  • Was your confidence in yourself affected by the other answers? Why?

Ask the group—

Q: In the second round, once you knew what was going on, what did you notice?
  • Think back to the first round—what did you observe then?

Q: What do you think you would have done if you were the real volunteer? Why?

Ask everyone—

Q: Do you think this has anything to teach us about the kind of influence we have on each other?
  • Do you think our potential to influence each other creates any responsibility to look out for each other? In what ways?
  • Can you see this principle at work in the sexual influence we have on each other? Talk about that.

To help students personalize the issue of sexual influence and responsibility, use **Line Up** (page 155 in this book) as a tool for group discussion or personal reflection.

WHAT'S MOST IMPORTANT?

The three levels of responsibility we all share: to God, to others, and to ourselves.

Read Mark 12:28-31 with your students, then use the following questions for discussion.

In this passage Jesus specifies the most important things in life. They parallel three levels of responsibility we have regarding our sexuality: to God, others, and ourselves. Two thousand years later, we have a responsibility to love all three: God, others, and ourselves.

YOU'LL NEED
- eight volunteers (see note below)
- pencils
- a sheet of paper on which you've drawn three different lines of different but similar lengths and labeled the three lines as "A," "B," and "C." Line B should be the longest, followed by Line A, with Line C as the shortest line.
- copies of **Line Up** (page 155), one per student

About the volunteers...
If your group is smaller, you can do the same thing with two or three setup volunteers and one real volunteer per round. In fact, you can play just one round if you need to.

If your students are using *What (Almost) Nobody Will Tell You about Sex*, you can direct them to **What's Most Important?** (page 85).

YOU'LL NEED
- copies of **What's Most Important?** (page 156), one per student
- pencils

If your students need some help, you could try pointing them to Psalm 139:13-16, Exodus 23:7, Proverbs 6:16-17, and Jeremiah 22:3.

Q: Jesus' use of the word *all* (or *holos* [HALL'-oss] in Greek) means *altogether, every bit*. Do you think it's possible to love God with all of you? Why or why not?
- How about others?
- What about yourself?

Q: How do you think people would treat each other romantically if they loved each other as they love themselves?

To help your students personally respond to the three levels of responsibility in this Mark passage, use the questions from **What's Most Important?** (page 156 in this book) as material for group discussion or personal reflection.

video-driven debate

ROE V. WADE

VIDEO

An honest look at the issues swirling around abortion.

Play the *"Roe v. Wade"* video and then ask the following questions:

Q: What is the one thing that stuck out to you most in this video?

Q: What did you agree with?
- What did you disagree with?

Q: In the video, some instances are offered where it would be okay to have an abortion, such as in the case of rape, or the health of the baby or mother, or if the child would otherwise grow up in poverty. How do you respond?

Q: Is it true, as was said in the video that girls who get pregnant get what they asked for? Why or why not?
- Do you think getting an abortion is more the pregnant woman's decision than the father's decision? Why or why not?

Q: Where do you think you got your ideas about abortion?
- Have your ideas grown or changed over the years? In what ways?

Q: What is your understanding of God's attitude toward abortion?
- What is your understanding of God's attitude toward those who have abortions?
- What is your understanding of God's attitude toward those who perform abortions?
- Can you support your understanding of these things from the Bible?

Q: Why do you think people get so emotional about abortion?

Q: How would you rate your emotional investment with regard to abortion?

I'm willing to die for my point of view because...	I don't feel like I have a settled point of view because...	I'm willing to kill for my point of view because...

Read the following arguments to your students.

FOR ABORTION	AGAINST ABORTION
• Laws against abortion kill women.	• Laws supporting abortion kill children.
• Legal abortions protect women's health.	• Legal abortions threaten children's health.
• A fetus is not a child until it is born.	• A fetus is an unborn child.
• Motherhood is a highly valued option for women.	• Motherhood is a woman's most important calling.
• Legal abortion supports a woman's right to choose.	• Legal abortion destroys an *unborn* woman's right to choose.
• Compulsory pregnancy laws are incompatible with a free society.	• Legalized abortion is incompatible with a free society.
• Outlawing abortion discriminates against those who have no voice in society.	• Legalized abortion discriminates against those who have no voice in society.
• Access to safe abortions is the law of the land.	• In this case, the law of the land is immoral.
• People who are against abortion should also be against war and capital punishment.	• People who are against war and capital punishment should also be against abortion.
• Abortion is birth control.	• Abortion is murder.
• Abortion is never wrong.	• Abortion is never right.
• Outlaw abortion and more children will bear children.	• Keep abortion legal, and more children will abort their children.
• The minority can't impose limits on the majority.	• Limits are necessary for democracy.
• Sometimes abortion is the only option.	• There's always another option.

Q: Which of these arguments is most compelling to you? Why?

Q: Which is most aggravating? Why?

Q: Do you think our group has a responsibility regarding abortion? Talk about that.

To help your students personalize the controversial issue of abortion, use the questions from **Roe v. Wade** (page 157 in this book) for additional group discussion or for personal reflection.

parent panel
THE HOME FRONT

Parents' perspectives about dating and sex.

Ahead of time, invite a few parents to be part of a parent panel. Ideally, these parents would be people your students respect—which, by the way, doesn't mean they need to be cool. You might want to give them these questions ahead of time so they can think about them and—if they wish—talk about their answers with their own children before they come to the group.

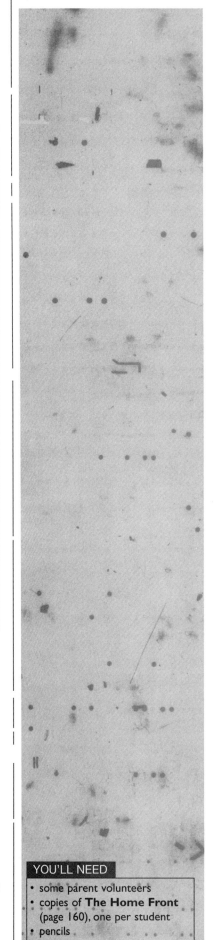

YOU'LL NEED
• some parent volunteers
• copies of **The Home Front** (page 160), one per student
• pencils

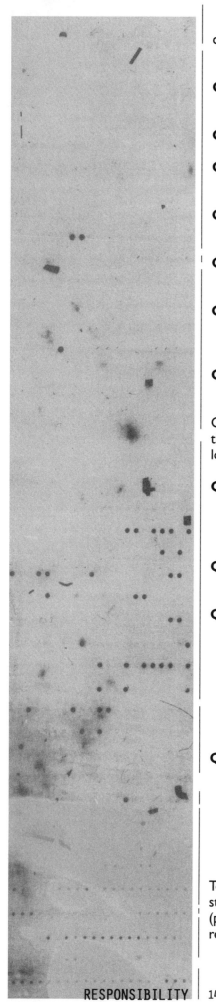

Let the panel know it would probably be best if they left before you lead a discussion with the group, but offer to tell them about it later if that's appropriate. Ask the parents these questions.

Q: Do you think it's different for teens today sexually than it was for you when you were young? Talk about that as personally as you can.

Q: What are your biggest fears about your kids' sexuality?

Q: How do your own sexual experiences affect how you approach your kids' sexuality?

Q: Without naming names, what mistakes have you seen other parents make in handling their kids' sexuality?

Q: Looking back, what do you wish you had done differently in addressing your own kids' sexuality?

Q: In Exodus 20:12 and then later in Ephesians 6:1-4, children are commanded to honor their parents. How do you like to be honored by your kids in the middle of what they're experiencing romantically and sexually?

Q: What do you think parents' responsibility is to their own kids when it comes to helping them figure out their sexuality?

Give students a chance to ask their own questions. Then thank the panel and excuse them, before debriefing the experience with your group. Ask your students the following questions:

Q: What's the most significant thing you heard from the parents' panel?
  • Why do you think that was significant?
  • Did you hear anything that was confusing? Troubling? Frightening? Angering? Surprising? Encouraging?

Q: Do you think sexual issues are different today than when your parents were young? Talk about that.

Q: Do you think parents should be concerned about what kids are going through sexually? Talk about that.
  • Without naming names, what mistakes have you observed parents making in handling their kids' sexuality?
  • Without embarrassing anyone, what mistakes have you observed kids making in responding to their parents' concerns about sexual issues?
  • Is there anything you wish you had done differently in communicating with your parents about dating or sex? Do you think you could revisit that now? Why?

Q: In Exodus 20:12 and Ephesians 6:1-4, we are given a clear picture of what it means to act responsibly toward our parents since we are commanded to honor them. How do you think you can honor your parents in the middle of what you're experiencing romantically and sexually?
  • What do you wish your parents understood about you and your dating life?
  • Why do you think people don't talk to their parents about dating and sex? Or is that just a stereotype?

To help students consider their parents and what they have contributed—and can still contribute—to their views of sex, use the questions from **The Home Front** (page 160 in this book) to guide additional group discussion or individual, personal reflection.

Openness versus isolation—and what we can do about it.

Read the following story aloud to your students.

YOU'LL NEED
- copies of **Alone Together** (page 161), one per student
- pencils

Here's what I wish I could take back...

I wish I could take back the silence. I wish I could take back the pretense that things were better than they were—that I was better than I am.

I'd been married four or five years, which made me some kind of expert to my friend who was just getting started. We went to lunch and talked about life in general. But there was something more on his mind. We were in the parking lot before he finally got it out. What he really wanted to talk about was a little sexual compulsion. It was nothing that can get a guy thrown in jail, he just expected it to go away when he got married. It didn't. So he felt confused and embarrassed and more than a little bit unfaithful to his bride. And he felt weak and alone because getting married was supposed to take care of such things. We all thought that in those days. It's what our fathers let us believe. I guess they were silent too.

My friend was embarrassed. He danced around the truth, trying to say it delicately. I was embarrassed too. But I hung in there, making a lot of eye contact, nodding as he spoke. I did everything I could to make him believe I understood his struggle. He thanked me when we said goodbye. I said I would pray for him.

What I didn't say was that I was wrestling with the same sexual compulsion. I stood there in a parking lot, listening and nodding and making my friend believe I understood—never once telling him why.

I was too ashamed of my own failure and, I suppose, startled by his openness. I was caught up in a false responsibility to be this guy's example or mentor or something. And then the moment passed and I was too embarrassed to back up in the conversation and tell the truth. So I didn't. I blew some smoke about praying for him, and I let him leave that conversation alone with his pain.

I left the conversation alone with my pain too—and with the realization that I was a liar.

If I could take that back, I think I would tell my friend, "Thanks so much for letting me into your struggle. That makes it easier for me to let you into mine, because I'm struggling with the same thing. Frankly, I thought I was the only one. I really hate it, but I don't know how to stop. Will you pray for me, because I'll sure pray for you. In fact I'd love it if you'd ask me how I'm doing with this about once a week. I think just knowing you're going to ask would help me."

I can't take it back. I haven't seen that guy for 20 years. The damage is done. I hope God was as persistent and generous with my friend as God was with me. Because eventually God helped me find a way of dealing with that sexual compulsion. But that's another story.

A few years ago, I tried to track down my friend. I didn't find him. I was surprised at how many men there were in that part of the country who have the same name. Here's what I wanted to tell him. I wanted to say, "I'm sorry I lied to you. I'm sorry I let you tell your story so honestly while I held on to my own story. Please forgive me. You were the better man that day."

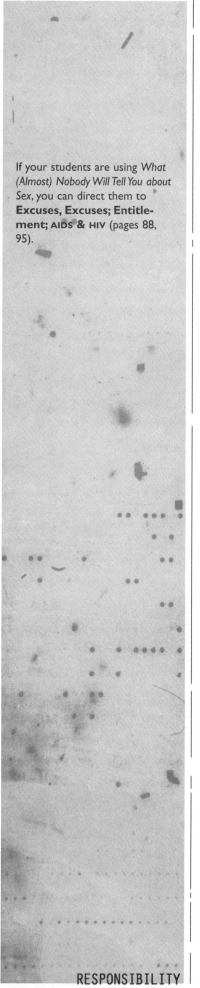

Q: Why do you think so many people live in isolation, thinking and feeling as though they are the only ones dealing with specific issues?
- Do you think there's any solution to that? What could one be?

Q: Someone has to go first. What do you think it takes to be that person?
- How does sharing with another person relate to our responsibility toward them?
- What do you think that costs?
- What do you believe it's worth? Why?

To help students further realize how their story might be shared, use the questions from **Alone Together** (page 161 in this book) for additional large or small group discussion, or possibly as a tool for individual, personal reflection.

If your students are using *What (Almost) Nobody Will Tell You about Sex*, you can direct them to **Excuses, Excuses; Entitlement; AIDS & HIV** (pages 88, 95).

U DA MAN!

Q: Is there any hint of David in you? Reflect upon that a bit.
- You probably haven't had anybody killed (if you have, maybe you should take that up with your youth worker before you go to bed tonight). But have you taken sexually what wasn't yours to take? Reflect on that a bit.
- Think for a moment—has God already sent Nathan to you in one form or another?
- If so, what happened?
- Could Nathan be in the wings, waiting for the right moment to tell you a story?

Look at Matthew 5:27-28.
Q: Does this passage speak to your situation today?

Write a letter to God about the condition of your heart. What do you need God to do for you now that you can't do for yourself?

DEAR GOD,

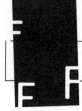

Reflect on these questions by yourself or with your group.

Q: Have you ever tried to help someone deal with a sexual issue or problem? How did it go?
- If you knew then what you know now, what would you have done differently?

Q: Has anyone ever tried to help you deal with a sexual issue? What did they do well?
- What do you wish they had done differently?

Q: Think about the people closest to you—parents, siblings, cousins, teachers, friends, neighbors, and pastors. What sexual issues do you think they could be going through now? What makes you think that?
- Do you think you have resources to help them (without harming you)?
- How do you think you might pray for them? What would remind you to pray for them?

TALK ABOUT IT

Reflect on these questions.

Take a few minutes and rate these people according to the following scale—

> 1—person you'd be most likely to talk to about the issue listed, if you ever struggled with it
> 2—person you'd be second most likely to talk to about the issue listed
> 3—person you'd be third most likely to talk to about the issue listed
> 4—person you can't imagine talking to about the issue under any circumstances.

	Mom/stepmom	Dad/stepdad	Sibling	Grandparent	Cousin	Aunt/Uncle
Compulsive masturbation						
Pornography						
Sexual fetish						
Pregnancy						
Peeping Tom voyeurism						
Nonstop fantasizing						
Sexual harassment						
Rape						
Sexual abuse						
Irresponsible flirting						

	Neighbor	Friend	Teacher	Pastor	Youth pastor	Therapist	Chat room acquaintance
Compulsive masturbation							
Pornography							
Sexual fetish							
Pregnancy							
Peeping Tom voyeurism							
Nonstop fantasizing							
Sexual harassment							
Rape							
Sexual abuse							
Irresponsible flirting							

Q: If you're as sick as your secrets, how sick are you?

☐ Nearly dead because...   ☐ I've been better because...   ☐ Couldn't be better because...

Q: Think back a year. Compared to then, how would you say you're doing these days?

☐ Much better because...   ☐ About the same because...   ☐ Falling apart because...

 (continued)

Reflect on these questions.

Q: What do you think would have to happen for you to be much better a year from now?

Q: Do you believe you have what that takes? If not, do you think you know where to get it?

Write or draw or encode the secret that makes you sickest.

Q: What does it cost you emotionally, spiritually, and relationally to keep that secret?

Q: Can you afford to keep paying that price?

Q: What do you think it would cost you to let someone in on your secret?
  • Which looks like the bigger price—keeping the secret or letting it go? Why?

LINE UP

Reflect on the questions.

Q: What people are the greatest influences on you? How do they influence you?

Q: Describe their influence—
- ☐ Positive because...   ☐ Neutral because...   ☐ Negative because...

Q: In several scientific studies, peer example has been a major force in teen sexual behavior. How does your own experience confirm or contradict this?

Q: What kind of influence do you think you have on others' sexual behaviors and attitudes?
- ☐ Positive because...   ☐ Neutral because...   ☐ Negative because...

Q: Why do you think that's true?

Q: How do you feel about that influence?

Q: Is there anything you wish you could change about the way others influence your sexual attitudes and behaviors? If so, what would that be?
- Why would you like to change that?
- Is there someone who can support you in that wish?

Q: Is there anything you would like to change about the way you influence other people's sexual attitudes and behaviors? If so, what would that be?
- Why is that important to you?
- Is there someone who can support you in that wish?
- How would you describe your desire for change if God happened to be listening right now (which, by the way, he is)?

WHAT'S MOST IMPORTANT?

Reflect on these questions by yourself or with your group.

Q: Which is most challenging for you: loving God with your heart, soul, mind, or strength?

☐ My heart because...   ☐ My soul because...   ☐ My mind because...   ☐ My strength because...

• Do you think any of these—your heart, soul, mind, or strength—affect your sexual experience more than the others?

Q: Think about someone you are interested in right now, or maybe even dating now. If you viewed them first as a brother or sister in Christ and then as a dating partner, do you think that might make a difference in how you think about them sexually?

• Do you think it might make a difference in the way you act toward them sexually? Why?

Q: Who do you think could give you some help in deepening your brother-sister perspective?

ROE V. WADE

Q: Describe your emotional reaction to the word abortion.
   • Why do you think you feel that way?

Q: How do you think your views on abortion compare with those of people at your school?
   • How do your views compare with those of people at your church or youth group?

Q: Maybe you've thought about having an abortion, maybe you've had one, maybe someone you've gotten pregnant had one, maybe you know someone who had one. Given all this, how has your own life been affected by abortion?

Q: Do you think you have any responsibility to act with regard to abortion? If so, what do you think you should do? Why?
   • What do you think you have to gain or lose by acting on your belief about abortion?

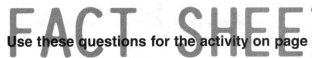

Use these questions for the activity on page

1. What percentage of Americans over the age of 11 show evidence of genital herpes?

   Over 20 percent—that's about one in five.

2. What percentage of sexually transmitted disease infections occur in people under the age of 25?

   About 66 percent—that's about two out of three.

3. What percentage of girls who get pregnant before age 18 earn a high school diploma by the age of 30?

   30 percent—and seven of 10 don't get a high school diploma at all.

4. What percentage of Americans are infected with HIV?

   About .003 percent—that's three of every 10,000.

5. What percentage of women infected by chlamydia don't know they're infected because they have no obvious symptoms?

   Up to 85 percent—that's almost nine out of 10.

6. What percentage of men infected by chlamydia don't know they're infected because they have no obvious symptoms?

   Up to 40 percent—that's four out of 10.

7. What percentage of people infected by chlamydia—who don't know they're infected because they have no obvious symptoms—are capable of infecting another person with the disease?

   100 percent—that would be 10 for 10 for those of you keeping score at home.

8. What percentage of people using condoms for contraception become pregnant within the first year of use?

   About 15 percent—more than one out of 10.

9. What percentage of adolescents who've had sexual intercourse are no longer sexually active?

   About 25 percent—about one in four stop soon after they start.

10. What percentage of American males and females ages 15 to 19 are still virgins?

    About 50 percent—that's one in two.

The average yearly wages of Americans without a high school diploma is $9,790.
—U.S. Census, 1990

There are approximately 272,639,608 Americans and about 900,000 of them are HIV positive.
—Medical Institute, 1998

Contact the Medical Institute for a cool video that covers these and other useful facts about sexual responsibility.

P.O Box 162306

San Antonio, Texas 78716

—Except where noted, numbers courtesy the Medical Institute (San Antonio, Texas).

THIS IS A TEST

Reflect on these questions by yourself or with your group.

Q: Is there anyone you know whom you fear may be infected by a sexually transmitted disease? If so, why do you think that may be true?
- How did you come to possess that knowledge?
- Knowing what you know, what are your options?
- Do you believe it's possible that person might go for a blood test if you offered to go along? Why?

Q: If you've been sexually active, how do you know you're not infected?
- Have you been tested since your last sexual contact?
- What do you think you have to gain or lose by getting a blood test?
- What do you think you have to gain or lose by not getting a blood test?

Q: What do you think is your responsibility to yourself and others when it comes to infectious diseases? Why? This is a test

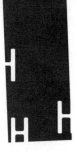

THE HOME FRONT

Refelct on these questions by yourself or with your group.

Q: How would you describe your relationship with your parents?
- Think back through the past year. Would you say your relationship seems better, worse, or about the same? Why?
- How do you think they would answer that question? Why?

Q: How comfortable do you feel talking with your parents about dating, love, or sex?
- ☐ Completely comfortable because—
- ☐ It depends because—
- ☐ Completely uncomfortable because—

Q: How comfortable do your parents seem to feel talking with you about dating, love, or sex?
- ☐ Completely comfortable because—
- ☐ It depends because—
- ☐ Completely uncomfortable because—

Q: What do you think it means to act responsibly and honor your parents in the middle of what you're experiencing romantically and sexually?
- How do you feel about that?
- Do you think there's anything you need to do over again with your parents?

ALONE?

Reflect on these questions.

Q: Do you feel isolated?

Q: Do you think you have the ability to go first and let out some of the issues that you are struggling with? Why?

Q: Do you think you have any responsibility to tell your story?
  • Are there circumstances in which you think it might be unwise to tell your story? Write down why.

Q: "We're only as sick as our secrets," the old saying goes. How sick are you?
  • Is there someone you trust enough to come out of your isolation a little bit? If not, would you be willing to ask God for such a friend? Would you be willing to start looking for that person?

CHAPTER 7

DO-OVERS

before you teach this lesson...

Sooner or later, everyone needs do-overs.

People who use sex as a weapon and people who've been hammered with sex. People who make bad choices and dumb mistakes. People whose sexual experiments blow up in their faces. People who know Mr. Lust is a natural born liar but believe him anyway (hey, maybe this time things will be different). People so arrogant or stupid they honestly believe they're not like the rest of us. People consumed by thoughts of the next orgasm and people consumed with pride because they've never had sex. People who wish they'd known back then what they know now. We know who we are.

Everybody—sooner or later—needs do-overs.

But can we get them?

Children learn about do-overs in friendly games of hopscotch or marbles. A do-over is a second chance when someone makes a mistake. It's a gift between friends. No one has a right to demand do-overs—no one can just say, "Shut up, I'm taking do-overs." A do-over is a favor, an act of grace. Grace is what this chapter is mainly about. Do-overs for people who commit sexual fouls—which is to say, all of us.

First, the bad news: for single people, young and old, sex is a high-risk behavior, like driving under the influence. If nothing goes wrong, maybe nobody gets hurt; if things go badly, maybe someone dies.

That worst-case scenario—someone dies—raises the stakes from, say, lying. Tell a lie and, if things go badly, the worst that happens—for you, at least—is you get caught and suffer the consequences of breaking trust. Unpleasant but probably endurable.

Getting caught sexually includes outcomes such as pregnancy and sexually transmitted infections.

A solo pregnancy is endlessly difficult no matter what. Ask around—you may find women making the best of hard situations, but you'll be hard-pressed to find a single mother who thinks she got away with anything.

Ditto sexually transmitted infections. At this writing, half a dozen epidemics run amok. They are unstoppable—there are treatments, but no cure.

Don't believe such things can happen to you? Please.

Getting caught sexually may also include unanticipated emotional consequences. There's an interesting idea in Paul's first letter to the Christians at Corinth: "Flee from sexual immorality," he says. "All other sins a man commits are outside his body, but he who sins sexually sins against his own body" (1 Corinthians 6:18). Sex has an unusually personal effect because it is uniquely *inside* rather than outside us; sex is not something we merely *do*.

This makes sense to anyone who's been surprised to find herself feeling shame about things she's done. Some people respond to those feelings by building up calluses where the pain is—like the tough spots on a tennis player's hands or a dancer's feet. But a lot of people decide it's just not worth it. According to the Medical Institute, one of every four adolescents who becomes sexually active stops soon after she or he begins. The good feelings they got from sex presumably didn't offset the bad feelings. The attachment they felt was nullified by the pain of separation. They gave it a shot—maybe more than one. But eventually it's like, why bother?

Which is too bad. Good sex is very good. It's not the meaning of life, but it's a good thing. It's sad when people get a bad impression of a good thing.

Do-overs are second chances for people who commit boundary violations. You can't demand do-overs, but God is awfully good about giving them. The trick is people giving do-overs to each other.

It's no secret that sex with the wrong person can be life-threatening.

All of which begs the question: Can 16-year-old boys and girls, burned out on premature sex, get do-overs? The answer depends on how we answer another question—Is God *for* us or *against* us?

If God is against us, it's Game Over, there won't be any do-overs. We'll die, forgiven but still guilty. Don't say God didn't warn us.

If, on the other hand, God is for us, there's hope. We still must contend with the natural consequences of our behavior, but there's supernatural hope. "There is," as Betsy ten Boom told her sister Corrie, "no pit so deep that God's love is not deeper still."

For people who grew up hearing about the irreversible effects of sexual failure—how much worse it is than other wrongs—this is hard to believe. But, if the Bible is true, this is also true: God's forgiveness covers every kind of wrong. Because God is gracious, people like us get a chance to begin again, starting right where we are, even though it's not where we're supposed to be.

Just to be certain we've said it, let's underscore one lonely group of folk who need do-overs in spite of themselves. They are the ones who were—or, God forbid, are—abused by their fathers, brothers, sisters, uncles, aunts, cousins, babysitters, teachers, pastors, and boyfriends (if we've left out anyone, it's only because we can't bear to go on).

These victims of sexualized violence—and it is violent, however silently it may creep—these victims tend to blame and punish themselves for what was done *to* them, not *by* them.

Michael Kelly Blanchard sings,

The trouble with me is I can't seem to trust.
My wounds just bleed and they won't heal up.
I don't know where I'd be if I'd never been touched.
But I know I don't like me much.

—"The Trouble with Me"
from the album *Be Ye Glad*, (Diadem Music)

That's as good a summary as you'll find this side of Tori Amos. The song ends with this meditation:

There is no sadness that God cannot feel
there is no sorrow that he cannot heal
moment by moment he's there where you hide
tenderly holding you close as you cry
Jesus the Lord of the lonely inside
Jesus the Lord of all love crucified

Hard as it may be to accept, these words point to the One who heals the broken-hearted and binds their wounds (Psalm 147:3). If we do nothing else with do-overs, let us offer sanctuary and hope to victims of sexual violence.

what's in this lesson...

reflect
a moment...

To help your students most effectively, you need to make every effort to process your own sexual experiences, questions, and struggles. Here are some questions to get you thinking:

Q: Describe your personal history with sexual do-overs.
  • Who else knows your history?

Q: Is there anything in your history that remains a closely guarded secret? Spend some time thinking, writing, or talking with someone about that.

Q: If you've been the victim or perpetrator of any form of sexual abuse, what did you do about that?
  • What remains to be done?

Q: Think for a moment about the people in your group. Do you have reason to believe any of them need sexual do-overs?

Q: Have you ever struggled over the concept of sexual do-overs? Spend some time thinking, writing, or talking with someone about that.

Q: Describe your current need for do-overs.
  • How did you reach this understanding?

Q: If you had just one hour to talk with kids about sexual do-overs, what would you try to communicate?
  • Why do you think that's so important?
  • How would you try to communicate during that hour?

In our own
words

— video opener
| DO-OVERS | —————————————————————— | VIDEO |

Introduce and show the video clip **"Do-Overs."** Then ask questions something like these.

Q: What strikes you as the most significant thing you heard in this video?
  • Why do you think that's important?

Q: Talk about anything that surprised you in the video.
  • What makes that surprising?

Q: Talk about anything that confused you in the video.
  • What's confusing about that?

Q: Do you believe these two really got do-overs from God? Why?

Q: Let's make up an ending for the guy's story.
  • Do you think he's over the pain of rejection? Why?
  • What do you think he'll do next? Why that?
  • If you were a close friend, what would you tell him?
  • How do you think it all ends? Why?

Q: Let's make up an ending for the girl's story.
  • Do you think she's had her chance at love and now it's over? Why?
  • What would you say to her if she were your friend?

If your students are using *What (Almost) Nobody Will Tell You about Sex*, you can direct them to **A Second, Third, and Sixty-Third Chance** (page 99).

YOU'LL NEED

- copies of **A Second, Third, and Sixty-Third Chance** (page 177), one per student
- pencils

Your Bible probably includes a note that this story is not in the earliest and best manuscripts. See William Barclay's comments on page 126 about this.

You may have already looked at this passage from a different perspective in **Boundaries**. For additional questions and further insight, see page 126.

A Sunday School teacher had just concluded her lesson and wanted to make sure she had made her point. She said, "Can anyone in the room tell me what you must do before you can obtain forgiveness of sin?" There was a short pause, and then, from the back of the room, a small boy spoke up. "Sin," he said.

Q: Listening to these two, what do you think about the possibility that you could get do-overs with God if you needed them?

word from God

A SECOND, THIRD, AND SIXTY-THIRD CHANCE

How Jesus treats sexual failures.

Read John 8:1-11 with your students.

> **Jesus was just hanging out one day when these religious folks decided to test him. They brought to him a woman in desperate need for a do-over. She had been caught in the midst of having sex with a married man. The law demanded that this woman be killed for her sinful act.**

Q: If you were going strictly by the rules, does this passage leave any question that the woman was guilty?

Q: How many times have you ever been caught doing something you knew deserved immediate punishment? A few times, huh?
- Have you ever been caught in act and dragged to "the authorities"?
- What was the outcome? Did you receive mercy or were you punished to the full extent of the law?

> **Jesus does a really interesting thing after this woman's accusers challenge him for an immediate verdict in this trial. He bends down and just starts writing in the sand. Wouldn't you love to know what he wrote? (I heard someone say once that they thought that perhaps Jesus was writing in the sand the names of the all the women the Pharisees and teachers of the law had slept with in the past.) The bottom line is that we do not know—but whatever he wrote sure freaked them out.**
> **Slowly, one by one, the Pharisees leave the scene after Jesus challenges them with the words, "Anyone here without sin can cast the first stone." The fact is, Jesus was the only one in that crowd who had the right to cast that stone. But he didn't, either.**

Q: Does this story give you reason to believe Jesus is for us or against us? Discuss that.

Q: Did this woman deserve a do-over? Why or why not?

Q: When we make mistakes regarding our sexuality, do we deserve do-overs?

Q: Why do we get them?

> **One of the last things Jesus says to this woman is, "I don't condemn you."**

Q: Do you believe most Christians feel they're in a place where they don't feel condemned by God when they mess up sexually?

Q: Do you believe you're in a place with God where you can say, "I don't feel condemned by him despite my sexual screw-ups"?

Q: How can we get to a place in our spiritual lives where feeling no condemnation from God is a regular part of our experience with him?

The last thing that Jesus says is, "Go now and leave your life of sin." Forgiveness and a do-over was offered to her on a plate. It was free of charge and available to her. All she had to do was receive it. But then Jesus goes on and says, "Hey, stop sleeping around." It seems that part of a do-over is the chance to get it right. Or in her case, using Jesus' language in the story, to stop getting it wrong.

Q: Why do you believe Jesus put that expectation on this woman caught in adultery? Why do you think Jesus commanded her to stop doing what she was doing?

Q: How hard is it to "just say no" to those things that have entrapped us in the past?

Q: What's your attitude about do-overs for people you know who take them for granted and make the same mistakes over and over again?

Q: If the woman had repeated her sin and been brought before Jesus again, what do you think he would have said to her?

To help students personalize God's willingness to let them have a do-over, use the questions from **A Second, Third, and Sixty-Third Chance** (page 177 in this book) as material for large or small group discussion or personal individual reflection.

the last word

case studies
WHO ME?

Common examples of folks who need do-overs and our own need for a fresh start.

There's a Spanish story about a teenage son who packed up and left home. He ran away, yet the father set off to find him. He searched for months to no avail. Finally, in a last desperate effort to locate him, the father put an ad in a Madrid newspaper. The ad read: "Dear Paco, meet me in front of this newspaper office at noon on Saturday. All is forgiven. I love you. Your Father." On Saturday 800 Pacos showed up, looking for forgiveness and love from their fathers.
—Bits and Pieces, October 15, 1992, p. 13

So many of us are looking for forgiveness. The fact is that we as Christians can find it in Jesus who sets us apart from the rest of humanity. Have a listen to some of these really difficult—yet true—stories of people who are in desperate need of do-overs, and then we'll discuss them together.

I guess it all started when I was about 12. My older brother got a copy of a porno magazine and hid it under his bed. One day I was searching for something and found it—it wasn't very well hidden. I had never seen anything like that in my life and I was blown away that women would allow themselves to be photographed in positions like this.

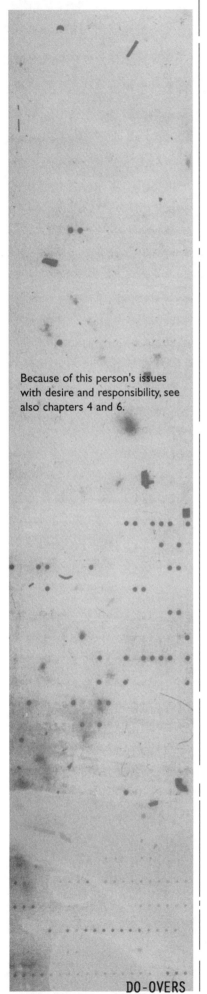

Because of this person's issues with desire and responsibility, see also chapters 4 and 6.

It started slowly at first—I would sneak into his room and just slowly go through all the pictures. I was a little grossed out in the beginning, but the more I looked at the magazine the more attractive it became to me. I can't really remember when it happened first, but I sure can remember how good it felt. Masturbating felt so good that all I could think about all day while at school was getting home to do it again. Here I am 12 years old and obsessed with these sexual feelings. Man they felt good.

I guess when I was about 14 those urges to want to masturbate got stronger and stronger. I remember once on a youth group trip to the beach those feelings got so strong inside me that I had to literally run into the bushes. At this point in my life I was masturbating sometimes up to four or five times a day—talk about a problem.

I'm twenty now. For about six years I've been seeking a solution to this problem, but nothing seems to be getting better. My stack of porno is so high I can barely see over it. There is a nude beach about 50 miles away from where I live, and I spend most weekends down there taking pictures when ladies are not looking. I hate what I do and who I am, but something just drives me to do this. I need help so bad, in fact, I wish I could just start all over again.

What a mess. Here's someone in desperate need of a do-over. The kind of do-over that only Jesus can give.

Q: Where do you think this person's problems first began? What could he have done about it back then to stop himself from getting in this huge hole?

Q: If this person came to you with this story of his life, what's the first thing you would tell him that he would need to do? What's the second? How about the third?

Q: From the sound of this person's account, do you think he feels the "no condemnation" that Jesus spoke about to the woman caught in adultery?

Q: How can this person get to a place where he believes Jesus doesn't condemn him for what's taking place?

Q: What do you believe Jesus' phrase "Go and sin no more" means here? What are some practical things that this person can do to make this command a reality?

This is so hard to talk about. I have never shared this with anyone before—it just makes me feel so dirty and abused. You'll have to bear with me as I tell my story—I have never done it before.

We were such a close family. I would stay over at my cousin's place down the road nearly as much as my own. My uncle seemed just as much my father as my own. Our families did everything together—vacations, field trips, barbeques—you name it. We loved each other so much.

That is, until my 15th birthday. I'd planned to spend this special night at my cousin's house—we were going to do a sleepover the way we'd done so many times before. My cousin fell asleep way too quickly that night—we had a lot more fun planned than what we actually did. I was a little bored now that she had fallen asleep so I went downstairs to watch a bit of TV.

This is the tough part. From seemingly nowhere my uncle came into the TV room and sat down beside me. I gave him a big hug as he wished me another happy birthday. What he gave me was the worst birthday anyone could ever have. I don't need to go into the details, do I? I suppose you can imagine what happened next. My favorite uncle forced himself on me in a way that is only designed for intimate married lovers. I tried to scream but he told me that he would tell everyone that I forced him to do it to me. Somehow back then that made sense...so I did nothing.

He is in jail now. I finally had the courage to come forward and tell my mom what happened. No one believed me at first. Perhaps that was one of the worst things about the whole situation. I can remember overhearing discussions my parents had about the possibility of me making this up. That really hurt. No one really believed me until my favorite cousin stepped up and shared with everyone that this had been happening to her for years.

It has been seven years since that night. I have never had a boyfriend and, truth be told, I hate men. Whenever I am touched by a man I feel filthy. All I can think about whenever a man approaches me is my 15th birthday. It wasn't very happy.

This is a really tough story to hear. Tough maybe because some of us in this room might be able to relate personally. Let's process what we've heard.

Q: A lot of people who go through times of sexual abuse feel guilty for what's happened. Why do you think this is?

Q: Although this woman was the victim, does she still need a do-over? Why or why not? If so, how might her do-over be different from her uncle's, if at all?

Q: What advice would you give a person that shared a story like this with you?

Q: What do you think Jesus would want to say to this lady?

It happened so quickly. He was my boyfriend for only a few weeks when we went on a special date. After dinner and a movie we went up to this special place that he had heard about. We were having such a good night and everything seemed to be going so well.

He parked the car and we could see the city lights spread out underneath us like a blanket. Believe me, romance was in the air. We started to make out a little, just gentle kissing really. As our kissing became a lot more enthusiastic, I could tell that he was becoming very excited. (Don't tell anyone, but I was too.)

He started to slip his hand under my blouse, and I tried to pull back. I never had had anyone touch me there before. My head was screaming at me to stop him from doing this, but my body was screaming just as loud to let it keep going. Before I knew what was happening, his other hand was grabbing downstairs, and I knew that at this point it just had to stop. I pushed him away with all my might and tried to get out of the car, but he jumped on top of me and locked the door.

Before I knew it, my skirt was lifted way up and his pants were down. It was impossible to resist—he was way too strong for me. It was over nearly as soon as it had begun. I wanted to be angry with him for what he had done, but you know what? I was a lot angrier with myself. Perhaps I shouldn't have worn this skirt, I thought to myself. Maybe Mom was right—it did send the wrong message. I did allow him to touch my breast, so surely the signal I gave to him was

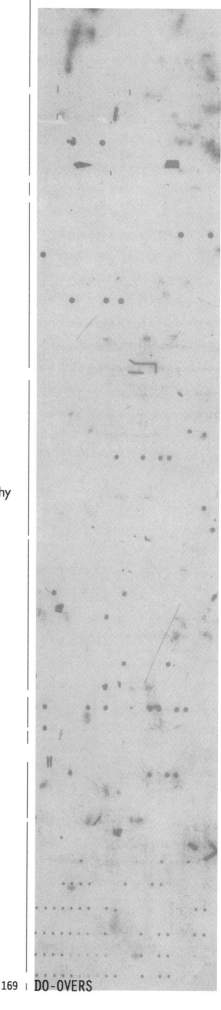

that I was willing for more.

Well, that was about a month or so ago. He has not called me since, and I have never told anyone. There was no way this was rape. Surely it could never be that if there was even a small part of me that wanted it to happen. I just can't believe I lost my virginity that way. I suppose there is nothing to stop me from having sex with anyone I'm attracted to now. It's not like I can regain my virginity and be pure for the man I'm going to marry, is it?

Q: Was this girl to blame in any way for what happened that night in the car? Why or why not?

Q: Do you think she's right? Is there no way it was rape? Why?

Q: What advice would you give this girl if she came to you and told this story?

Q: How important is it for her to not feel condemnation for what has happened? Is it possible for her to forgive herself for what she perceives is something that she let happen? How can she do this?

Q: An important issue in this story is the feeling that she can never regain her purity. Is this true? How does your answer relate to the kind of do-overs that Jesus offers?

The point in interacting with these stories is to see how important the need is for do-overs in our lives. We all need them at one point or another, and Jesus can come through with them no matter how messed up the situation appears. We need to learn how to trust and believe that do-overs are free gifts from God, given so we can live lives that honor him.

Q: What is the one thing you're going to take home from this discussion? Can you share that with the person sitting next to you?

Q: We all need do-overs at some point and I am betting a bunch of you need them now. What can we do as a community of people who love each other to help each other receive do-overs from Jesus?

To close this meeting I would like you to get in groups of three or four with the same gender and share with each other—in as little or as much detail you like—an area where you need a do-over. Be as honest as you can. If you feel like you need additional help, please let me know that after we're done here. After you share, spend some time praying for each other, focusing specifically on asking God that you would be free from condemnation for this stuff and that you might be able to receive your very own do-over. Let me remind you of our agreement to keep things shared in this room appropriately confidential. Do you have any questions about confidentiality? Okay, let's take about 10 minutes to share and pray.

For more information on confidentiality, see page 25.

Listen to the buzz and time this as loosely as you wish.

In other words

video opener —
LES MISERABLES ———————————————— VIDEO

Do-overs give fresh starts.

The movie, *Les Miserables*, is based on the novel by Victor Hugo. In this clip you will see Jean Valjean (jon val-jon—use your best French accent—played by Liam Neeson), just released from prison, on his way to report to his parole officer. He's told he cannot sleep on the street, so he finds a meal and a bed at the home of a bishop. In the middle of the night Jean wakes and steals the bishop's fine silver. He's caught by the police, and what happens next is a remarkable example of a do-over. Instead of turning him in, the bishop tells the police he gave this man all the silver and, in fact, he forgot to take the candlesticks. He experiences forgiveness and is given an opportunity to leave the past behind and start over.

Introduce the video clip and show it to your students.

YOU'LL NEED
- TV or video projection unit
- VCR or DVD player
- *Les Miserables* video, cued to the clip, beginning 3 minutes after the Columbia logo ("You can't sleep here"), ending 6½ minutes later ("And now I give you back to God")

Q: If you had been the bishop, what do you think you would have said when the police brought the man back with the stolen silver?

Q: Obviously this ex-prisoner did not deserve the type of do-over that the bishop gave him. Why do you think the bishop showed such remarkable grace?
- How do you think you would have felt if you were the man?

Q: If you had been the bishop, what would you have hoped the man would now do with his life?

Q: Can you think of any other examples of incredible do-overs in real life, books, or movies? Describe what happened and discuss whether or not the people involved deserved that do-over.

Q: Can you think of a time when you ever got a do-over or an unexpected gift of grace?

As we're going to see, it's part of who God is to give us do-overs when we mess up.

small-group Bible study
SCARLET LADY

The profile of a person who got serious do-overs from God.

If your group is largish, break it into teams of half a dozen with the following assignment.

I'd like each group to read Joshua 2:1-21, Joshua 6:20-25, Hebrews 11:31, and James 2:25. Then write a "Once upon a time..." story about Rahab, including what you take to be the moral of the story. In about 15 minutes, I'll ask you to read your story to the rest of us.

Do everything you can to ensure that each group receives wild applause for its efforts.

Q: What do you think is the most important thing that comes out of Rahab's story? Why do you think that's important?

Q: Why do you think God works with people like Rahab? Why not a queen or a Joan of Arc type? Why the proprietor of a whorehouse?

Look at 1 Corinthians 1:26-31 with your students.

Q: How does this passage relate to the story of Rahab?

To help students further personalize the story of Rahab and apply it to their lives, use the questions from **Scarlet Lady** (page 178 in this book) in large and small group discussions, or as a tool for individual reflection.

If your students are using *What (Almost) Nobody Will Tell You about Sex*, you can direct them to **Scarlet Lady** (page 106).

YOU'LL NEED
- Bibles
- pencils
- paper
- copies of **Scarlet Lady** (page 178), one per student

For variety, assign one or more groups to the same task with Hosea 1:1-9 and 3:1-5.

If your students are using *What (Almost) Nobody Will Tell You about Sex*, you can direct them to **Jesus, the Unexpected** (page 108).

YOU'LL NEED

- copies of **Jesus, the Unexpected** (page 179), one per student
- pencils

> The acceptance of oneself is the essence of the whole moral problem and the epitome of a whole outlook on life. That I feed the hungry, that I forgive an insult, that I love my enemy in the name of Christ—all these are undoubtedly great virtues. What I do unto the least of my brethren, that I do unto Christ. But what if I should discover that the least amongst them all, the poorest of all the beggars, the most impudent of all the offenders, the very enemy himself—that these are within me, and that I myself stand in need of the alms of my own kindness—that I myself am the enemy who must be loved—what then? As a rule, the Christian's attitude is then reversed. There is no longer any question of love or longsuffering. We say to the brother within us, "Raca," and condemn and rage against ourselves. We hide it from the world; we refuse to admit ever having met this least among the lowly in ourselves.
>
> —Carl Jung,
> *Modern Man in Search of a Soul*
> *(Harcourt Brace and World Harvest Books)*

If your students are using *What (Almost) Nobody Will Tell You about Sex*, you can direct them to **Calling Your Bluff** (page 101).

YOU'LL NEED

- copies of **Calling Your Bluff** (page 180), one per student
- pencils

---

another Bible study
JESUS, THE UNEXPECTED

How Jesus feels about people who love him—no matter where they came from.

Read Luke 7:36-50 with your students, then use the following questions for discussion.

> **Put yourself in the scene in Luke 7:36-50 as, say, a waiter. You go into the kitchen, shaking your head. The cook asks, "What? Is something wrong with the food?" "Nope," you say, "the food is great, but there's this woman out there—"**

Q: Pick up the story from there—what would you tell the cook you saw and heard?

> **So, the cook saunters through the dining room. He comes back shaking his head. He says, "I don't know this Jesus character, but I sure recognize the hooker. Isn't he an evangelist or something? I mean, what is he thinking!"**

Q: What do you tell him?

Q: How long do you think Jesus would last on the staff of a local church or Christian organization? Why?

Q: How long do you think the local church or organization you're thinking about would last if they didn't get rid of Jesus fast?

Q: How long do you think it would take the woman in this story to fit in at that local church? Why?

Q: Do you think most Christians really believe Jesus when he says things like he said about—and to—this woman? Talk about that.

To help your students identify further with the characters in this biblical narrative, use the questions from **Jesus, the Unexpected** (page 179 in this book) to guide additional group or individual reflection.

---

another Bible-driven discussion
CALLING YOUR BLUFF

One way God uses sexual failures to accomplish higher purposes.

Read John 4:1-42 with your students, then use the following questions for discussion.

Q: Why do you suppose Jesus struck up a conversation with this woman?
- What do you think he had to gain or lose by talking with her?
- What do you think she had to gain or lose by talking with him?

Q: Why do you think the insight Jesus had into this woman's life grabbed her attention so dramatically?
- Why do you think the people in town reacted so strongly to her claim that she met a man who told her everything she ever did?

Q: Have you ever seen God use this kind of messenger to reach people? If so, can you tell us the story?

> **Here's what it looks like from here. It looks like forgiven people come in two flavors:**

1. Those who feel so grateful to be forgiven that they stop judging other people and—like Jesus—become the frien of sinners.

2. Those who seem to feel like they somehow deserved to be forgiven—some kind of exemption for special people, perhaps. So they become very hard to live with because they're always pointing their finger at people who do bad things or fail to do good things.

Is it just me or does it look that way to you as well? Let's talk about that.

Q: Which kind of Christian do you want to hang with? Why or why not?
- How do you think people become the kind of Christian you want to hang with?
- How do you think people become the other kind of Christian?
- What do you think we can do to encourage each other to become the best sort of forgiven people?

To help students further appreciate the do-over Jesus gives to the woman in John 4, use the questions from **Calling Your Bluff** (page 180 in this book) as a springboard for additional group discussion or individual reflection.

┌─ another great Bible study! ─
│ FALLING...AND BOUNCING BACK │
└─────────────────────────────

Exploring truth, consequences, repentance, and restoration.

Before your read the psalms, review the story of David's great fall and recovery in 2 Samuel 11 and 12.

Q: What do you think David was experiencing, thinking, or feeling as he went through these events?

lust	foolishness	stupidity
deceit	love	treachery
hope	frustration	grief
remorse	arrogance	guilt

Q: Have you ever seen these processes at work in someone you know? If so, talk about what you saw, but without incriminating anyone.

Read Psalms 32 and 51 with your students, then use the following questions for discussion.

Q: What stands out for you in these songs? Why do you think that's important?

Q: Do you believe David is sincere? Why or why not?

Q: At what point in the story do you imagine David wrote these songs?

Before Nathan intervened because—	When Nathan intervened because—	When the baby was sick because—	After the baby died because—	Some other time because—

Q: Have you ever felt any of the emotions in these songs?
- If so, can you talk about that?

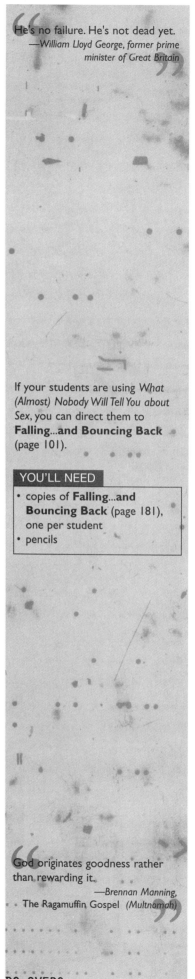

"He's no failure. He's not dead yet.
—William Lloyd George, former prime minister of Great Britain"

If your students are using *What (Almost) Nobody Will Tell You about Sex,* you can direct them to **Falling...and Bouncing Back** (page 101).

YOU'LL NEED
- copies of **Falling...and Bouncing Back** (page 181), one per student
- pencils

"God originates goodness rather than rewarding it.
—Brennan Manning, The Ragamuffin Gospel (Multnomah)"

Q: What would you say David learned from his wrongdoing and God's forgiveness?
   • To what extent would you say you've learned those lessons?

| I get it completely because... | I still have a lot to learn because... | I don't get it at all because... |

To help students more personally apply Psalms 32 and 51 to their own lives, use **Falling...and Bouncing Back** (page 181 in this book) as a tool for individual personal reflection.

another Bible-driven discussion
CRAVING SALT

Hunger for that old life.

Here's some background on Genesis 18 and 19—
It seems like whatever happens, God helps Abraham. As the fortunes of everyone around him rise and fall, Abraham grows more prosperous. When Abraham gets in trouble—even when it's his own fault—God rescues him. It's a remarkable relationship. Lot, on the other hand, has always acted like a bum. Now—when there's about to be big trouble in Sodom and Gomorrah—God chooses to let Abraham in on it.

Read Genesis 18:20-19:29 with your students, then use the following questions for discussion.

Q: Why did the Lord tell Abraham what he was going to do with Sodom and Gomorrah?

Q: God seems mighty angry with Sodom and Gomorrah. Why do you think he was?

Q: Lot seems to me like a real loser. I mean, what kind of a guy would offer his two daughters to an angry mob so they can rape them?

Q: When Lot and his family were escaping God's judgment on Sodom and Gomorrah, Lot's wife turned around to have a look at the fireworks display and then got turned into a pillar of salt for her trouble. Why did God do that to her?

I read this story recently about a guy in college who was a believer but kept talking about his old life before he met Christ. He seemed to dwell on the past so much that his friends ended up nicknaming him "Salty" in honor of Lot's wife. I think the reason she was turned into a pillar of salt was because her heart longed to be back in that place.

Q: Do you sometimes feel yourself looking back at your old life and how fun it would be to be back there?

Q: How do you think God feels about that?

Q: Why do some of us have the tendency to look back at our lives before we met Jesus, or maybe at the lives of our friends who are not believers, and secretly long to do the things we once did or that our friends do?
   • What do you think God would say about that?

YOU WANT ME TO MARRY A WHAT?

How far is God willing to go to prove his love? Farther than you might think.

Read Hosea 1-3 with your students, remembering that Judah and Israel are split into two kingdoms. Then use the following questions for discussion.

Q: What do you think God is up to here, in big-picture terms?
- How do you think the prophet Hosea fits into the deal?

Look at Leviticus 21:7-15 with your students.

Q: What do you think went through Hosea's mind when God asked him to do something that would get him fired if he were a priest?
- What do you think went through Gomer's mind when God's prophet popped the question?
- What do you think went through people's minds when the wedding announcement appeared in the paper?

Q: Try to put yourself in Gomer's shoes. How do you think she felt when her husband bought her at an auction?
- What does this tell you about God and do-overs?
- Where do you imagine this family story goes from here?

They all live happily ever after because—	They struggle but pull through because—	Gomer goes back to her old ways because—	Hosea can't forget his shame and punishes Gomer because—

To help students further understand God's purpose in the story of Hosea and Gomer, use **You Want Me to Marry a What?** (page 182 in this book) as material for more group discussion or individual reflection.

THE FIRST AMENDMENT

The freedom that can come after deep sexual pain.

"If we claim to be without sin," John says, "we deceive ourselves and the truth is not in us. If we confess our sins, he is faithful and just and will forgive us our sins and purify us from all unrighteousness" (1 John 1:8-9).

That's what this is about. We'll take the next 15 minutes [or whatever length of time you think is appropriate in your group] **to reflect on where we've caused or experienced sexual pain, or both. We're starting from where we *are*, not where we're supposed to be.**

Write, draw, sculpt, draw on the butcher-paper graffiti wall—do whatever makes sense to you as a way to describe or picture your own wrongdoing or the wrong that has been done to you. If you feel the need to keep your reflections private, you're welcome to do so. There's an area for private reflection in that corner of the room [or next door or whatever makes sense].

You ready? I'll mark time about every five minutes.

When you think people are finished or it's time to move on, give everyone a chance to look at what's been publicly displayed. (If there is only one story displayed and

---

If your students are using *What (Almost) Nobody Will Tell You about Sex*, you can direct them to **You Want Me to Marry a What?** (page 108).

YOU'LL NEED

- copies of **You Want Me to Marry a What?** (page 182), one per student
- pencils

YOU'LL NEED

- paper
- pencils
- pens
- markers
- butcher paper
- Play-Doh
- tape (optional)
- whatever else you can pull together that's artsy
- copies of **The First Amendment** (page 183), one per student

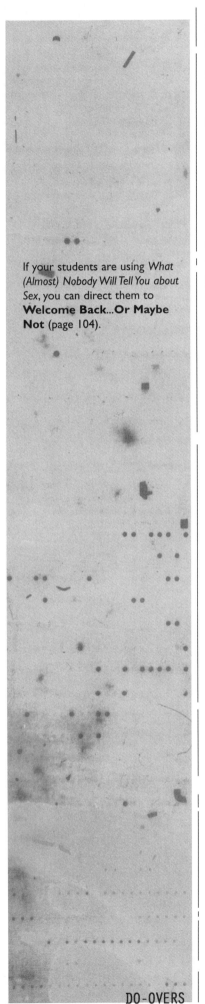

everyone else chooses to keep their expressions private, this can still be a remarkable experience.)

Q: What was it like for you to express your sexual reality over the last few minutes? Talk about that.

Q: Based on this process, do you think you have any unfinished business? Can you talk about that?
- What do you think you need to do next?
- What help do you think you could use?
- How do you think God wants to be involved in this process?
- What do you think you may have to gain or lose by getting help?
- How can we pray for you?

To help students more fully realize their freedom in Christ, use the questions from **The First Amendment** (page 183 in this book) for additional group discussion or individual reflection.

If your students are using *What (Almost) Nobody Will Tell You about Sex*, you can direct them to **Welcome Back...Or Maybe Not** (page 104).

A SECOND, THIRD, AND SIXTY-THIRD CHANCE

Read John 8:1-11. Then reflect on these questions.

Q: What stands out for you in this story?
  • Why is that important to you?

Q: Does it feel more normal for you to treat people the way Jesus treated the woman caught in the act of adultery or the way her accusers treated her?

Q: While Jesus doesn't condemn her, he does make it clear that he wants her to stop her adultery. What does that tell you about Jesus' view toward you when you sin?

Q: Do you know anyone who's becoming a better person because he's getting sexual do-overs? Reflect on that a bit.

Q: Do you know someone who could use sexual do-overs now?

Q: And you? How easy is it for you to believe Jesus might really give you do-overs when you need them most?

Write a brief letter to God about your need to give or get sexual do-overs.

DEAR GOD,

SCARLET LADY

Look at Joshua 2:1-21, Joshua 6:20-25, Hebrews 11:31, and James 2:25.
Reflect on these questions.

Q: What do you learn about God in these passages?
 • Why do you think that message stands out for you?

Q: Are there any ways in which you're like Rahab? Reflect on that a bit.
 • Are there ways in which God is treating you like he treated Rahab? Reflect on that a bit.

Q: If the story of Rahab demonstrates how God accepts people, what do you want to do in response?

JESUS, THE UNEXPECTED

Read Luke 7:36-50. Then reflect on these questions.

Q: What do you think is the most important thing in this story? Why do you think it's important?

Q: With whom do you most closely identify in this story?
- Simon the Pharisee because...
- The woman because...
- Jesus because...
- The other guests because...

Q: Do you think a person has to be a hooker to appreciate how much she's been forgiven?

Q: How do you think you do at treating people as if Jesus were really serious about this?
- ☐ Not well at all because...
- ☐ I could do better because...
- ☐ I do pretty well most of the time because...

Q: How well would you say you do at treating yourself as if Jesus were really serious about this?
- ☐ Not well at all because...
- ☐ I could do better because...
- ☐ I do pretty well most of the time because...

Q: What do you think you may have yet to really learn from this story?
- What do you imagine you have to gain or lose by learning that lesson?

Write a note to God about that.

DEAR GOD,

CALLING YOUR BLUFF

Read John 4:1-42. Then reflect on these questions.

Q: What stands out for you in this story? Why is that significant to you?

Q: What do you have in common with this woman?
  • How are you different?

Q: Would you consider what you've done, or failed to do, to be any worse (or better) than the woman in this story?

Q: Can you imagine using your story of failure to introduce people to Jesus? Reflect on that a bit.
  • What do you think you have to gain or lose by using your failure story to introduce people to Jesus? Is it worth it? Why or why not?

FALLING AND BOUNCING BACK

Read Psalms 32 and 51. Then reflect on these questions.

Q: What stands out for you in these passages?
- Why do you think that strikes you?

Q: With what do you most closely identify in the songs?

Q: In what ways do you think you are least like David? Why?

See if you can write a poem or draw a picture that describes how you feel about God's intervention in your most significant failure.

> God uses all the wrong roads to bring us to all the right places.
> —C. S. Lewis

Q: Have you yet made the kind of recovery David made? Reflect on that a bit.
- What do you think you need to do to have that kind of recovery?
- How do you think God might fit into your recovery?

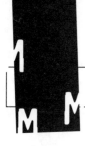

YOU WANT ME TO MARRY A WHAT?

Read Hosea 1-3. Then reflect on these questions.

Q: How do you respond to the story of Hosea? Reflect on that a bit.

Q: If you were Hosea's friend, and he told you what he thought God was asking him to do, what would you have told him? Why?
- If you were Gomer's friend, and she told you she was going to marry the prophet, what would you have told her? Why?

Q: The prophets often seemed to be God's stuntmen—doing outlandish things to make big points for people who didn't seem to be getting the picture. Has God done something spectacular to get your attention?
- Do you know anyone you think could stand to hear the story of Hosea and Gomer (and God and his people)? If so, what makes you think that person needs to hear this story? What do you think you can do about that?

THE FIRST AMENDMENT

Reflect on questions.

An old preacher said—

"You will know the truth and the truth will make you flinch before it sets you free."

Q: Have you been flinching about the truth of your sexual behavior? Write about that.

Q: How close to sexually free would you say you are right now?

❑ Knocking on the door because...   ❑ Well on my way because...   ❑ Not even close because...

• What do you think it will take to get you where you need to be?
• How does God fit into your answer above?
• Who else can help?
• What do you think you want to do about that?
• Is there anything keeping you from it?

Plumbing and Wiring:
FAQs

Don't hate us. We didn't ask the questions. We're just trying to respond honestly to the questions teens ask. So skip the ones you think are obvious and just be glad there's somebody out there who knows less than you. Feel free to circle whether you knew it or didn't know it.

Q: How do people learn to kiss?
The truth is that kissing comes pretty naturally to a girl and a guy. Sometimes noses get bumped and braces get locked up, but those mishaps are rare.
knew it/didn't know it

Q: How do people breathe when they kiss?
Although girls' and guys' mouths are pretty preoccupied during kissing, their noses usually aren't—they do the work for them.
knew it/didn't know it

Q: What exactly happens during sex?
The sexual act proceeds through several phases. The first is an excitement phase, marked by an increase in pulse and blood pressure as blood rushes to the surface of the body. Genital fluids are also secreted during the excitement phase. The penis becomes erect, and the vagina expands. The second phase is the plateau phase, which is pretty brief and may conclude with an orgasm. The third phase is the resolution phase where the body functions return to normal.
knew it/didn't know it

Q: What is an orgasm?
An orgasm, also called a *climax*, is the peak of physical sexual excitement and gratification. Physically, it's marked by a faster pulse, higher blood pressure, and muscle contractions in the penis and vagina. Sperm ejaculates from the penis. An orgasm is marked by an overwhelming feeling of pleasure and release.
knew it/didn't know it

Q: Does an orgasm always happen during intercourse?
Not always. Sometimes two people will feel fairly aroused and have a grand ol' time together, but neither will have an orgasm. It's also possible to have an orgasm before or after sexual intercourse.
knew it/didn't know it

Q: Is an orgasm different for a guy than for a girl?
Well, yes, because they have different body parts. Both experience quick, rapid muscular contractions, but the female's orgasm usually lasts longer. Another bonus for the female is that she can often have several orgasms in succession, while the male usually has one. However, one bonus for the male is that since he usually becomes more quickly aroused, he has orgasms more consistently during sexual intercourse.
knew it/didn't know it

Q: Do orgasms always feel the same?
No, an orgasm almost always feels good, but sometimes it feels great. How great relates to how emotionally connected you are to the other person,

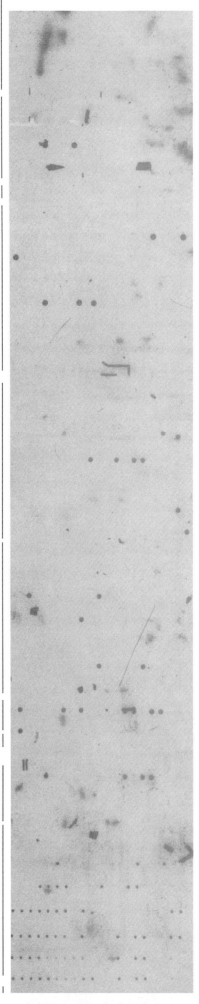

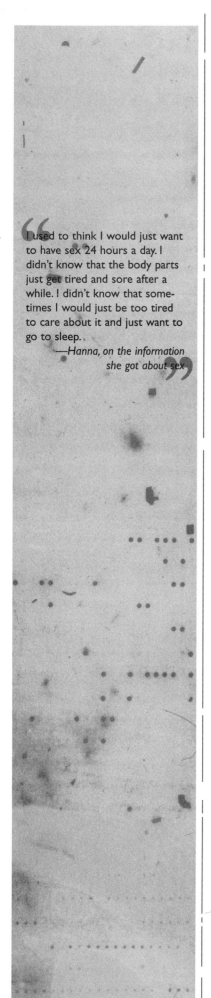

how physically tired and aroused you are, how mentally distracted you are, and how comfortable you feel to enjoy what's going on.
knew it/didn't know it

Q: How long does an orgasm last?

Although the orgasm is the most talked-about phase in sexual intercourse, it's actually short, ranging from five to 30 seconds.
knew it/didn't know it

Q: What's an erection?

When a male becomes sexually aroused, the blood flow into his penis is increased and the blood flowing out of his penis is temporarily reduced. As a result, the tissue swells, and the penis enlarges, hardens, and elevates.
knew it/didn't know it

Q: I've heard that alcohol will help your sex drive, but I've also heard it will hurt it. What's the deal?

Alcohol is a depressant, so it tends to reduce inhibitions and dull decision-making skills. So people who've had something to drink may become more flirtatious or willing to try things they wouldn't even consider when sober. Because of this, some people jump to the conclusion that alcohol increases sex drive. But actually alcohol depresses the nervous system and diminishes muscular coordination and nerve sensation. Sober sex is generally more pleasurable than sex under the influence. Perhaps the biggest gotcha is that the risk of pregnancy and contracting sexually transmitted infections increases with carelessness, so reread the first sentence and do the math.
knew it/didn't know it

Q: Does sex hurt?

It can hurt—especially the first few times and especially for women. Imagine going dancing for the first time. Since you don't know what you're doing—and you haven't practiced—you might hurt yourself or the other person. The same is true for sex when you're new at it. This is one reason your patient, caring, committed partner (by which we mean *spouse*) can make the experience go more smoothly. This is especially true when you both believe practice makes perfect.
knew it/didn't know it

Q: Does the size of the penis matter?

Most males assume the average size of an erect penis is 6 inches, and then they get worried because theirs is smaller than that. But the reality is that an erect penis measures around 5.1 to 5.2 inches, and a nonerect (or flaccid) penis measures 3.5 inches. Regardless of the penis size, the male doesn't need to worry about it. The female's body adjusts to fit whatever size he is.
knew it/didn't know it

Q: Is masturbation wrong?

Ah, that's a biggie. Masturbation, or stimulating your own genitals, is pretty controversial. Some Christians believe it's wrong all the time, others believe it's right almost all of the time—and still others fall somewhere in the middle, arguing that it's okay to do periodically as long as it isn't associated with lustful fantasies or doesn't become a preoccupation (which it tends to become the more you do it). You might want to talk to a parent or Christian adult

you respect to get some more guidance. There's more about masturbation in **Desire** (page 104).
knew it/didn't know it

Q: What is oral sex?
Contrary to what some may think, *oral* sex is not *talking about* sex. Instead, it means using the mouth to stimulate another person's genitals.
knew it/didn't know it

Q: Is oral sex the same as sex?
By definition, no (in the sense that babies can't be born from oral sex). But don't forget that sexually transmitted infections can be contracted through oral sex and that it's way past the line of what you want to be doing before marriage.
knew it/didn't know it .

Q: What if my breasts are different sizes?
That's not uncommon. There's nothing wrong with it, especially when your breasts are still developing. However, if you notice any breast lumps, you should have a doctor examine you just to make sure the lumps aren't tumors or cysts.
knew it/didn't know it

Q: What if my testicles are different sizes?
That's not uncommon. If the larger testicle is hard, you should have it checked by a doctor to make sure it's not a cyst, tumor, or hernia.
knew it/didn't know it

Q: What are wet dreams, and why do they happen?
Wet dreams are also known as nocturnal emissions. Starting at puberty, as a male's body goes through all sorts of changes, he's likely to have some fluid ejaculation from his penis. This usually happens at night and is often during a sexually stimulating dream—hence the term *wet dream*.
knew it/didn't know it

Q: Have I done something wrong if I have a wet dream?
Some guys feel guilty about wet dreams—maybe because it reminds them of wetting the bed or because they're dreaming about specific women. But it's really just a subconscious and natural event that doesn't necessarily mean anything.
knew it/didn't know it

Q: If the penis is withdrawn before ejaculation, can pregnancy still occur?
During extended foreplay, a small amount of preejaculatory fluid seeps from the penis. This fluid contains live sperm that can cause pregnancy. Because of this, withdrawing the penis from the vagina before ejaculation is not generally considered a safe form of birth control.
knew it/didn't know it

Q: And what exactly is foreplay?
Foreplay is the early stage of sexual "play" that gets a couple ready for intercourse. In other words, making out is foreplay.
knew it/didn't know it

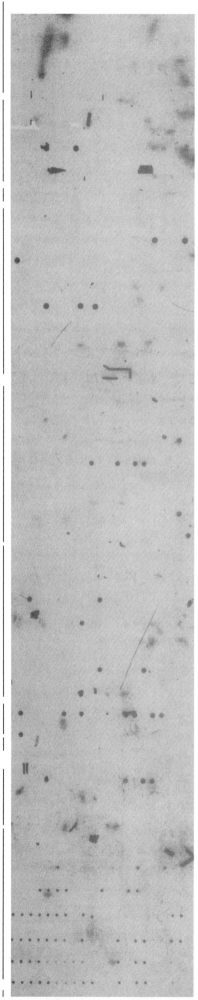

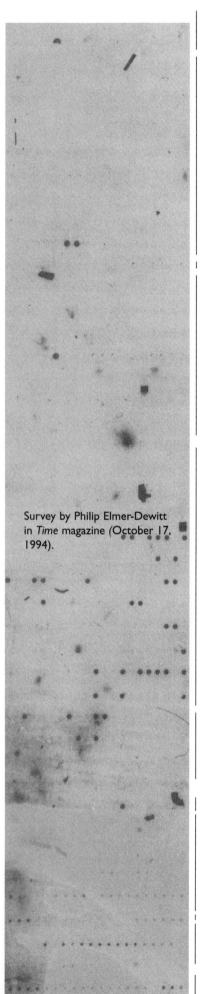

Survey by Philip Elmer-Dewitt in *Time* magazine (October 17, 1994).

Q: I've heard that a female won't get pregnant if she has sex standing up or if she has sex in a hot tub. Is that true?

A female can be jumping up and down, doing handstands, or doing cartwheels; but if she's having sex, she could get pregnant. The position doesn't matter, and neither does the environment. She can be in a hot tub, sauna, or even a waterbed—if she's having sex, she could get pregnant at any time.

knew it/didn't know it

Q: Does having sex change you physically?

For women the hymen (a membrane just inside the vagina) can break, which might hurt and cause some bleeding. If you get pregnant, there are *lots* of physical changes. For men nothing really changes physically, but either gender can pick up sexually transmitted infections—even from having sex only once. Oh yeah, did we mention that if you're a woman, you could get pregnant? Or that if you're a man or woman, you could get HIV? We don't mean to harp, but those are pretty huge deals.

knew it/didn't know it

Q: Sex is always neat and clean in the movies—is that right?

Sex is messy—not gross necessarily, but messy. When the male ejaculates, the two to six milliliters of semen containing about 300 million sperm have to go somewhere. Plus the vagina builds up additional lubrication. You figure it out.

knew it/didn't know it

Q: Christians are so prudish. They must have lousy sex, right?

Actually, quite the opposite is the case. One national survey of 3,500 Americans ages 18 to 59 (conducted by the University of Chicago in 1994) revealed that Protestant Christian women are most likely to achieve orgasm each and every time they have vaginal intercourse. Could this be a fringe benefit of following God's plan?

knew it/didn't know it

Back-to-basics biology

This is a cheat sheet on basic sexual biology. Use it to refresh your memory from health class. (This will not be on the test.) Feel free to circle whether you knew it or didn't know it.

ACCESSORY ORGANS—Sperm cells aren't capable of self-movement until ejaculation, and they're activated by seminal plasma fluid secreted by the prostate gland, ejaculatory ducts, seminal vesicles, and bulbourethral glands. These organs are important even though they can't be seen.
knew it/didn't know it

CERVIX—The opening from the vagina into the uterus, located at the far (internal) end of the vagina.
knew it/didn't know it

CLITORIS—The only organ in the human anatomy designed solely for sexual stimulation, the female clitoris is a two- to three-centimeter funnel loaded with nerve endings. It's very sensitive both to pleasure and pain.
knew it/didn't know it

CORONAL RIDGE—The bulge near the end of the penis is called the coronal ridge.
knew it/didn't know it

GLANS (OR HEAD)—If a male has been circumcised, the glans is visible at the end of the penis. If a male hasn't been circumcised, the glans is covered with loose skin called the **foreskin**.
knew it/didn't know it

LABIA MAJORA—The outermost ridges of the vulva designed to protect the rest of the vagina. If a female hasn't given birth, the outer lips of the labia majora probably meet at the center of her genitals.
knew it/didn't know it

OVARIES—The ovaries are female internal organs shaped like large almonds. They are located on either side of the uterus and produce some of the sex hormones that affect the menstrual cycle. But their primary function is to release one of about 400,000 eggs for reproduction 14 days before menstruation begins. The egg is either fertilized by a male's sperm and implants itself in the uterus, or it's discharged from the body with the menstrual blood flow. This process begins in puberty and continues until menopause.
knew it/didn't know it

PENIS—The penis is the external male organ for sexual intercourse and introduces sperm into the vagina. During sexual excitement, blood is temporarily trapped in the chambers of the erectile tissue in the penis, causing the penis to become enlarged, firm, and erect.
knew it/didn't know it

SCROTUM—A pouch in the male genital anatomy that holds two glands called the testes.
knew it/didn't know it

Information adapted from these resources:

• Clifford and Joyce Penner, *The Gift of Sex: A Christian Guide to Sexual Fulfillment* (Word Books, April 1982).

• *Encyclopaedia Britannica CD 98.* Encyclopaedia Britannica.

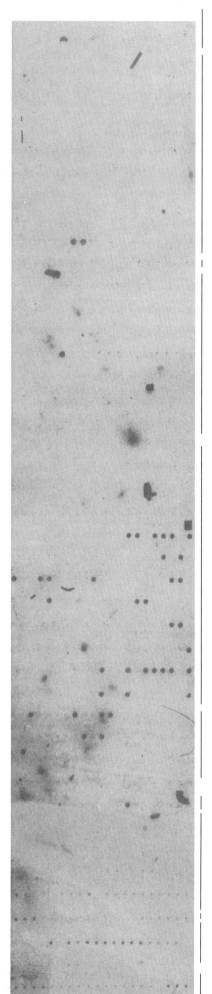

SHAFT—The cylindrical structure of the penis.
knew it/didn't know it

SPERM—Cells from a male that are capable of fertilizing a mature egg in the female reproductive system. The process of sexual arousal and ejaculation activates the otherwise immobile cells so they become self-propelled in the seminal fluid by means of a tiny tail that whips from side to side. Sperm are available more or less on demand in quantities of around 300 million cells per ejaculation. Under favorable conditions sperm live about three days after ejaculation.
knew it/didn't know it

TESTES—The testes (the primary male reproductive organ) are two small glands that move around in the scrotum and generate sperm.
knew it/didn't know it

UTERUS (WOMB)—A pear-shaped muscular organ in the female reproductive system, located between the urinary bladder and rectum and connecting through the cervix to the vagina. The lining of the uterus, the endometrium, secretes fluids that keep eggs and sperm alive and nourish fertilized eggs. If a mature egg isn't fertilized, it's flushed out with the endometrium through the vagina during menstruation.
knew it/didn't know it

URETHRA—A thin tube that carries urine from the bladder out of the body. In the male, the urethra also carries sperm from the seminal vesicles out through the penis.
knew it/didn't know it

VAGINA—A tube-shaped canal that leads from outside the body to the uterus, adapts in size to receive the penis during intercourse and expands to accommodate a baby during delivery.
knew it/didn't know it

VULVA—The external female genitalia that surround the opening to the vagina.
knew it/didn't know it

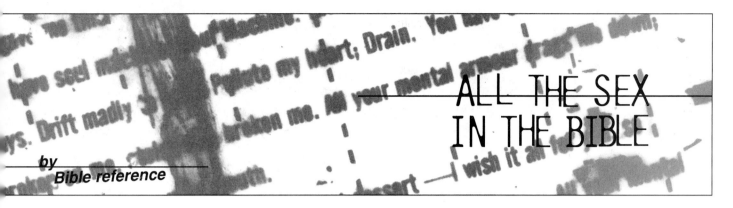

ALL THE SEX IN THE BIBLE

by
Bible reference

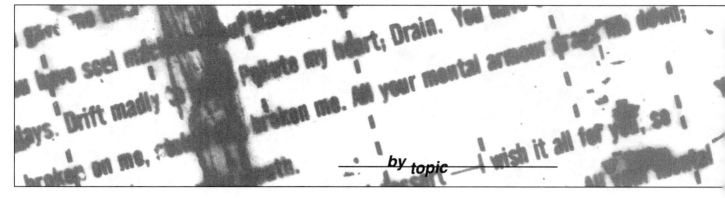

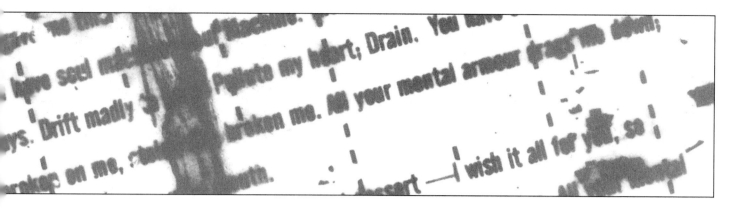

RESOURCES FROM YOUTH SPECIALTIES

Youth Ministry Programming

Camps, Retreats, Missions, & Service Ideas
(Ideas Library)
Compassionate Kids: Practical Ways to Involve Your
Students in Mission and Service
Creative Bible Lessons from the Old Testament
Creative Bible Lessons in 1 & 2 Corinthians
Creative Bible Lessons in John: Encounters with Jesus
Creative Bible Lessons in Romans: Faith on Fire!
Creative Bible Lessons on the Life of Christ
Creative Bible Lessons in Psalms
Creative Junior High Programs from
A to Z, Vol. 1 (A-M)
Creative Junior High Programs from
A to Z, Vol. 2 (N-Z)
Creative Meetings, Bible Lessons, &
Worship Ideas (Ideas Library)
Crowd Breakers & Mixers (Ideas Library)
Downloading the Bible Leader's Guide
Drama, Skits, & Sketches (Ideas Library)
Drama, Skits, & Sketches 2 (Ideas Library)
Dramatic Pauses
Everyday Object Lessons
Games (Ideas Library)
Games 2 (Ideas Library)
Games 3 (Ideas Library)
Good Sex: A Whole-Person Approach to
Teenage Sexuality & God
Great Fundraising Ideas for Youth Groups
More Great Fundraising Ideas for Youth Groups
Great Retreats for Youth Groups
Holiday Ideas (Ideas Library)
Hot Illustrations for Youth Talks
More Hot Illustrations for Youth Talks
Still More Hot Illustrations for Youth Talks
Ideas Library on CD-ROM
Incredible Questionnaires for Youth Ministry
Junior High Game Nights
More Junior High Game Nights
Kickstarters: 101 Ingenious Intros to Just
about Any Bible Lesson
Live the Life! Student Evangelism Training Kit
Memory Makers
The Next Level Leader's Guide
Play It! Over 150 Great Games for Youth Groups
Roaring Lambs
So What Am I Gonna Do with My Life?
Leader's Guide
Special Events (Ideas Library)
Spontaneous Melodramas
Spontaneous Melodramas 2
Student Leadership Training Manual
Student Underground: An Event Curriculum
on the Persecuted Church
Super Sketches for Youth Ministry
Talking the Walk
Videos That Teach
What Would Jesus Do? Youth Leader's Kit
Wild Truth Bible Lessons

Wild Truth Bible Lessons 2
Wild Truth Bible Lessons—Pictures of God
Wild Truth Bible Lessons—Pictures of God 2
Worship Services for Youth Groups

Professional Resources

Administration, Publicity, & Fundraising
(Ideas Library)
Dynamic Communicators Workshop for
Youth Workers
Equipped to Serve: Volunteer Youth Worker
Training Course
Help! I'm a Junior High Youth Worker!
Help! I'm a Small-Group Leader!
Help! I'm a Sunday School Teacher!
Help! I'm a Volunteer Youth Worker!
How to Expand Your Youth Ministry
How to Speak to Youth...and Keep Them Awake
at the Same Time
Junior High Ministry (Updated & Expanded)
The Ministry of Nurture: A Youth Worker's Guide
to Discipling Teenagers
Purpose-Driven Youth Ministry
Purpose-Driven Youth Ministry Training Kit
So That's Why I Keep Doing This! 52 Devotional
Stories for Youth Workers
Teaching the Bible Creatively
A Youth Ministry Crash Course
The Youth Worker's Handbook to Family Ministry

Academic Resources

Four Views of Youth Ministry & the Church
Starting Right: Thinking Theologically about
Youth Ministry

Discussion Starters

Discussion & Lesson Starters (Ideas Library)
Discussion & Lesson Starters 2 (Ideas Library)
EdgeTV
Get 'Em Talking
Keep 'Em Talking!
Good Sex: A Whole-Person Approach to Teenage
Sexuality & God
High School TalkSheets
More High School TalkSheets
High School TalkSheets from Psalms and
Proverbs
Junior High TalkSheets
More Junior High TalkSheets
Junior High TalkSheets from Psalms and Proverbs
Real Kids: Short Cuts
Real Kids: The Real Deal—on Friendship, Loneliness,
Racism, & Suicide
Real Kids: The Real Deal—on Sexual Choices, Family
Matters, & Loss
Real Kids: The Real Deal—on Stressing Out, Addictive
Behavior, Great Comebacks, & Violence
Real Kids: Word on the Street

Unfinished Sentences: 450 Tantalizing Statement-
Starters to Get Teenagers Talking & Thinking
What If...? 450 Thought-Provoking Questions to
Get Teenagers Talking, Laughing, and Thinking
Would You Rather...? 465 Provocative Questions
to Get Teenagers Talking
Have You Ever...? 450 Intriguing Questions Guarante
to Get Teenagers Talking

Art Source Clip Art

Stark Raving Clip Art (print)
Youth Group Activities (print)
Clip Art Library Version 2.0 (CD-ROM)

Digital Resources

Clip Art Library Version 2.0 (CD-ROM)
Ideas Library on CD-ROM
Youth Ministry Management Tools (CD-ROM)

Videos & Video Curricula

Dynamic Communicators Workshop for
Youth Workers
EdgeTV
Equipped to Serve: Volunteer Youth Worker
Training Course
The Heart of Youth Ministry: A Morning with
Mike Yaconelli
Live the Life! Student Evangelism Training Kit
Purpose-Driven Youth Ministry Training Kit
Real Kids: Short Cuts
Real Kids: The Real Deal—on Friendship, Loneline
Racism, & Suicide
Real Kids: The Real Deal—on Sexual Choices, Fan
Matters, & Loss
Real Kids: The Real Deal—on Stressing Out, Addi
Behavior, Great Comebacks, & Violence
Real Kids: Word on the Street
Student Underground: An Event Curriculum on
the Persecuted Church
Understanding Your Teenager Video Curriculum

Student Resources

Downloading the Bible: A Rough Guide to the
New Testament
Downloading the Bible: A Rough Guide to the
Old Testament
Grow For It Journal
Grow For It Journal through the Scriptures
So What Am I Gonna Do with My Life? Journalin
Workbook for Students
Spiritual Challenge Journal: The Next Level
Teen Devotional Bible
What (Almost) Nobody Will Tell You about Sex
What Would Jesus Do? Spiritual Challenge Journ
Wild Truth Journal for Junior Highers
Wild Truth Journal—Pictures of God